Purpose in Life

Kendall Cotton Bronk

Purpose in Life

A Critical Component of Optimal Youth Development

Springer

Kendall Cotton Bronk
Ball State University
Muncie
USA

ISBN 978-94-007-7490-2 ISBN 978-94-007-7491-9 (eBook)
DOI 10.1007/978-94-007-7491-9
Springer Dordrecht Heidelberg London New York

Library of Congress Control Number: 2013946046

Printed on acid-free paper

Springer is part of Springer Science+Business Media (www.springer.com)

Dedicated to CBB, CJB, and LCJB who imbue my own life with a deep and inspiring sense of purpose.

Foreword

As a human concern, purpose has been around at least as long as any of the world's great religions or philosophies. Whenever someone asks a deeply searching question such as "why am I here?", "what's the reason for my existence?", "what is my life about?", or "how can I make the best use of my time on this planet?", the concept of purpose inevitably arises. Finding purpose in life is a pursuit that links people of all historical epochs, social-cultural backgrounds, economic circumstances, and geographical settings. It is a timeless, universal feature of human experience.

Purpose also is an especially timely pursuit, in our day of dynamic global transformation. Technological change, as many commentators have pointed out, is "disrupting" practically every pattern of commercial and social existence. It seems as though nothing can be taken for granted any longer. Vocations that were once highly stable are disappearing, declining, or morphing into barely recognizable versions of their former selves (consider the present directions of journalism, law, medicine, education). Families are becoming dramatically more varied in their compositions as well as in their formation and duration. People are moving away from home communities with ever more expansive horizons in mind; and, in accord with this expansion, friendships and other intimate relations have gone global and virtual, with cell phone conversations replacing face-to-face encounters, social media replacing cell phone conversations, and who knows what replacing social media in the next technological revolution to come. Amidst all this sweeping alteration in everything that anchors a personal identity, it is little wonder that people are looking around for a compass to guide them through life. Purpose is such a compass *par excellence*—and, predictably, our mass media are full of stories about the value of purpose for success, health, and happiness in these often-perplexing times.

Despite the timeless and timely status of purpose as a core element of human experience, the scientific study of purpose has been surprisingly thin until very recently. This is not unusual in the human sciences, which tend to focus on narrower constructs that may be examined under controlled conditions in laboratory settings. Purpose is a sweeping, far-horizons type of goal that comes into play over extended periods of time in the crucible of major life decisions. To study it in a serious way requires exactly the kinds of methodological treatments prominent in the present book: deep, probing interviews; case studies of exemplary persons; and considerations of actual contexts that elicit purpose. Only a mature science can tackle a complex subject such as purpose with a range of methods suited to its complexity. The appearance of *Purpose in Life: A Critical Component of Optimal Youth Development* is a welcome sign that the psychological science of human development has reached this level of maturity.

Beyond its importance to psychological science, this book addresses a timely educational concern. The most pressing problem in education today is a shortfall in student motivation. This shortfall is not confined to disadvantaged neighborhoods or poorly-run classrooms (although it leads to especially damaging outcomes in such settings). Even in the best schools there are many students who find little meaning in their studies. Some of these students may grind out their work dutifully but without interest, getting by with whatever minimum grades the need to keep out of trouble; others shirk their academic assignments entirely. When young people spend countless hours, days, and weeks on activities that they find meaningless, there are psychological costs. I documented some of these costs in *The Path to Purpose*: they may include boredom and apathy, a debilitating anxiety, or an ensnarement in the lures of hedonism and cynicism. Unmotivated students are often the ones who are most"stressed out" in school, even though they are not often those who are working the hardest. The students who have found purpose in their schoolwork, in contrast, usually gain so much satisfaction from their efforts that long hours fly by without much anxiety. Working hard is not the problem: rather, the problem is working without knowing why, working without a clear purpose. For a young person, purpose is critical to enduring academic motivation.

The importance of purpose continues throughout life, and as people transition from one age to the next, they are often called upon to redefine themselves and their broadest goals. Doing so successfully is essential for health, happiness, and meaning. For this reason, people of all ages have much to learn from the scientific study of purpose. *Purpose in Life: A Critical Component of Optimal Youth Development* offers valuable information to scientists, educators, and people interested in the essentials of human development. Its author, Kendall Cotton Bronk, was a key player in our own early forays into the study of youth purpose at Stanford University. Now, with this book, she has shed bright new light on this key topic, a significant contribution to scholarship and practice alike.

Stanford, CA William Damon
March 2013

Contents

1 Introduction and Definition 1
History of the Purpose Construct 1
Defining Purpose 4
Philosophical Underpinnings 8
Purpose in Theories of Optimal Development 9
The Nature of Purpose 13
Scope and Outline of the Book 14
References 16

2 Measuring Purpose 21
Surveys Aligned with Frankl's Conception of Purpose 21
Ryff's Purpose in Life Sub-Scale 29
Antonovsky's Sense of Coherence Survey 30
Survey Measures of Meaning and Constructs Related to Purpose 32
Less Commonly Used Survey Measures of Purpose 33
Interview Protocols 36
Other Measures of Life Purpose 37
References 42

3 The Role of Purpose in Optimal Human Functioning 47
Stress 49
Coping and Substance Abuse 53
Psychological and Physical Well-being 54
Purpose and Health Behaviors 58
Other Positive Correlates of Purpose 60
References 63

4 Purpose across the Lifespan 69
Childhood 69
Adolescence and Emerging Adulthood 71
Midlife 79
Late Adulthood 81

Purpose Across the Lifespan 83
References 85

5 **Origins of and Supports for Purpose** 91
Evolutionary Basis for Purpose 91
Developmental Origins of Purpose 93
Opportunities and Experiences that Foster Purpose 94
Social Supports for Purpose 96
References 105

6 **Inspiring Types of Purpose** 109
Religious Purposes 113
Familial Purpose 118
Professional Purposes and Callings 119
Artistic Purpose 121
Civic and Political Purpose 122
References 125

7 **The Experience of Purpose Among Diverse Groups** 129
Affective Experience of Purpose 129
Social Experience of Purpose 132
Self-Focused Experience of Purpose 133
The Experience of Searching for Purpose 134
Experience and Prevalence of Purpose
Among Different Groups of People 136
References 140

8 **Exemplar Research** 145
Definitional Matters 145
Youth Purpose Exemplars 147
Purpose Development and Identity Formation 152
Youth Purpose Development 155
References 159

9 **Future Directions for Purpose Research** 163
Survey Measure of Purpose 163
Longitudinal Investigations 164
Investigations of Immoral or Ignoble Purposes 165
Role of Negative Experiences 166
Purpose among Youth From Highly Challenging Backgrounds 167
Different Types of Purpose 168
Cultural and Cross-cultural Studies 169
Physical Benefits of Purpose 170
Support for the Development of Purpose 171
References 173

Chapter 1
Introduction and Definition

> The truth is that as the struggle for survival has subsided, the question has emerged—survival for what? Ever more people have the *means* to live, but no *meaning* to live for.—(Frankl 1979, p. 21, emphasis added).

The question Frankl poses above is a timely and important one. What is the purpose of life? It is a question most people ponder at some point in their lives, so it is not surprising that significant bookstore shelf space is typically dedicated to tomes on the topic. However, the vast majority of these books are based on one person's theory, experience, or untested approach to discovering purpose. Given the growing psychological attention paid to the purpose in life construct, surprisingly few resources exist that outline the science behind it. What do we know about purpose, and how do we know it? What exactly is purpose, how do people discover it, and what difference does it make? This book is dedicated to synthesizing theoretical and empirical research that addresses these questions and others on the topic.

However, before launching into a discussion of that research, it is important to outline the conception of purpose on which the existing research relies. Similarly, it is important to understand where this conception originated. Therefore, this book opens with a definition of purpose and a discussion of the history of the construct.

History of the Purpose Construct

Researchers in psychology have been slow to recognize the importance of purpose to well-being (Van Dyke and Elias 2007), but Viktor Frankl (1959) was not. Frankl suffered greatly as a concentration camp inmate during World War II. He was subjected to 3 years of slave labor, torture, starvation rations, and other harsh indignities. But he survived, and he credited his survival to his ability to maintain an enduring and personally meaningful purpose. In fact, throughout his ordeal, Frankl recognized that among those individuals who were given the chance to survive, it was those who held onto a positive vision of the future who were the most likely to live. Individuals who maintained hope of reuniting with loved ones, or who had projects they felt they needed to complete, or who maintained a deep spiritual

K. C. Bronk, *Purpose in Life*, DOI 10.1007/978-94-007-7491-9_1,

faith—in other words individuals committed to various purposes—were the ones who most often endured. At the end of World War II, Frankl was freed from the concentration camp, and he wrote *Man's Search for Meaning* (1959) in which he detailed his experience as inmate #119104 and outlined his theory and approach to therapy based on the importance of discovering purpose.

According to Frankl, all individuals are capable of finding meaning, even in seemingly meaningless situations. Some influential philosophers, including French existentialists Sartre and Camus, believed that life had no meaning but that human beings needed to lead meaningful lives; therefore these philosophers argued that individuals *gave* their lives meaning. They *chose* or *selected* a meaning for their lives (Fabry 1988; Yalom 1980). Frankl, on the other hand, maintained that purpose and meaning existed, and individuals needed only to *discover* it. Just as the air is full of musical sound waves, meaning and purpose are all around us. However, to hear the music, individuals need to turn on the radio. Similarly to discover meaning in the world around us, people need to "tune in" (Fabry 1988, p. 4).

Freud believed the desire for pleasure was our greatest incentive for behavior. According to Adler, it was the desire for power. But Frankl believed meaning was our most powerful motivator (Frankl 1984). Pleasure and power, he maintained, are possible by-products of purpose, but purpose is neither a by-product nor a means to an end. Purpose or meaning—Frankl used these terms interchangeably—represents our ultimate goal, and discovering a purpose enables people to endure hardships and overcome negative states.

Frankl was the first individual to argue that because pursuing a personally meaningful purpose represents the foundation of human motivation, serious psychological problems can result from purposelessness. Frankl pointed to the consistent relationship between meaninglessness and hatred, boredom, criminal behavior, addiction, and depression. He argued that people often try to fill the void left by a lack of meaning with hedonistic pleasures, the pursuit of power, materialism, and neurotic obsessions and compulsions (Frankl 1984). Without purpose, existential frustration, often in the form of boredom, depression, and apathy, results. While a lack of purpose may not lead to psychopathology for all individuals, Frankl argued, for many it does. In fact, Frankl estimated that approximately 20 % of the psychological and psychiatric patient population and more than half of the general population suffered boredom and "existential frustration" associated with a lack of purpose in life (Crumbaugh 1977; Crumbaugh 1968; Crumbaugh and Maholick 1964).

As a result of Frankl's belief in the power of purpose, when he was released from the concentration camp he developed a therapeutic approach to counseling that seeks to help patients discover a purpose for their lives. Called Logotherapy, this meaning-centered approach is based on the assumption that all people are capable of identifying a reason for living, and that doing so helps individuals overcome negative states and live more fulfilling lives (Crumbaugh and Henrion 2001).

The idea that something as ethereal as a life purpose could influence one's behavior or motivation was counterintuitive to the prevailing wisdom of the time. Behaviorism and psychoanalytical theories, the prevalent approaches to human behavior at the time, viewed belief systems such as these as mere by-products of more fundamental human drives (Damon et al. 2003). Frankl disagreed adamantly with these propositions:

> Man's search for meaning is a primary force in his life and not a "secondary rationalization" of instinctual drives. This meaning is unique and specific in that it must and can be fulfilled by him alone; only then does it achieve a significance which will satisfy his own *will* to meaning. There are some authors who contend that meanings and values are "nothing but defense mechanisms, reaction formations and sublimations." But as for myself, I would not be willing to live merely for the sake of my "defense mechanisms," nor would I be ready to die merely for the sake of my "reaction formations." Man, however, is able to live and even to die for the sake of his ideals and values! (Frankl 1984, p. 99)

Logotherapy is based on the principle that having a reason or purpose for living is necessary for a fulfilling life (Frankl 1984; van Deurzen-Smith 1997). It is based on several key assumptions (Schulenberg 2004). The first is the Freedom of Will assumption, which means that although people cannot always control what happens to them, they can always control how they respond to the events in their lives (Crumbaugh 1971; Melton and Schulenberg 2008). The second is the Will to Meaning assumption, which implies that people's primary motivation is the desire to find meaning or purpose for their lives (Crumbaugh 1971; Frankl 1984; Melton and Schulenberg 2008; van Deurzen-Smith 1997). When the Will to Meaning is interrupted or blocked, existential frustration results (Frankl 1984). The last significant assumption is that life is inherently meaningful under all circumstances, even those involving unavoidable suffering and torture (Frankl 1984). Frankl believed that even helpless victims in hopeless situations could find meaning by choosing to live with dignity and by rising above the circumstances. He experienced this way of life firsthand as a concentration camp inmate.

As a first step to helping patients through Logotherapy, Frankl designed a set of rather informal questions, The Frankl Questionnaire, which he used to evaluate the degree to which his patients maintained a meaningful purpose (Crumbaugh and Maholick 1967). The questionnaire included questions such as *Do you feel that your life is without purpose?*

While Frankl was interested in the concept of purpose from a clinical rather than an empirical perspective, the broader psychological community took interest in his book, and Crumbaugh and Maholick, two researchers who worked closely with Frankl, used his informal questionnaire as the basis of their more rigorous 20-item survey called the Purpose in Life (PIL) test (1964; 1967). Most early empirical studies of purpose rely on Crumbaugh and Maholick's PIL, (Crumbaugh and Maholick 1967; Crumbaugh 1968). A fuller discussion of this and other influential measures of purpose can be found in Chap. 2 ("Measuring Purpose").

As a result of Frankl's writing and the newly created PIL test, psychological research on the purpose in life construct peaked for the first time in the 1960s. However, following that decade, the number of empirical studies conducted on purpose decreased, and it was not until the early 2000s that psychological research on the construct increased again, this time in conjunction with the emergence of the positive psychology movement (Seligman and Csikszentmihalyi 2000; Sheldon and

King 2001). Though Frankl focused on negative associations of purposelessness, consistent with the positive psychology paradigm, more contemporary researchers have increasingly focused on the positive associations of purposefulness.

Defining Purpose

Before outlining the ways in which purpose figures into positive psychology models and frameworks, it is important to be clear on what constitutes purpose. As with any emerging construct, theoretical conceptions and definitions of it varied in the past. Purpose has been regarded as key to decision-making (Maddi 1998), as an evolutionary adaptation (Boyd 2009; Klinger 1998), as a means of making sense out of chaos (Korotkov 1998), and as an individual's ultimate aim or goal (Damon 2008; Emmons 2005). Frankl (1959) described purpose as "inner strength" (p. 80),"the responsibility which a man has for his existence" (p. 80), "the 'why' of [one's] existence," (p. 101), "the specific meaning of a person's life at a given moment," (p. 110), and "[that which] life expected from us" (p. 108). Early research on the topic utilized the definition of purpose put forth by Frankl (1959) and operationalized by Crumbaugh and Maholick (1964; 1967) as "*the ontological significance of life from the point of view of the experiencing individual*" (p. 201). In other words, purpose refers to a subjective sense of one's life as meaningful. Other researchers have emphasized specific aspects of purpose or meaning, including a cognitive component (e.g. a belief that one's life is meaningful), an affective component (e.g. a feeling that one's life is meaningful), and a motivational component (e.g. a striving for meaning in one's life; Wong 1998). However, most definitions of purpose, both historical and contemporary, feature three key elements: commitment, goal-directedness, and personal meaningfulness.

According to Erikson (1968; 1980), commitment, the first critical component of purpose, is an important aspect of healthy human development in general and of positive identity development in particular. In order to establish a coherent sense of self, individuals need to commit to certain beliefs, values, and orientations to establish a coherent and unified sense of self. Adolescents, Erikson noted, begin to make "choices and decisions which will, with increasing immediacy, lead to a more final self-definition, to irreversible role pattern, and thus to commitments 'for life'" (1980, p. 119). In the same way, individuals must be able to identify some aim to which they are willing to commit their time, resources, and mental energy (Bronk 2012; Damon 2008; Damon et al. 2003). Without this commitment a purpose in life, which is enduring by nature, cannot be established.

A commitment to something is necessary for goal development, and a purpose in life is a goal of sorts. Goal-directedness represents the second aspect of the definition of purpose. Ryff and Singer (2008) identify individuals with high levels of purpose in part by their "having goals and directedness;" Benard (1991) likewise highlights the role of "persistence" and "goal-directedness" in purpose; Yalom (1980) notes that purpose refers to "an intention, aim, function" (p. 423); and Baumeister (1991) notes that purpose is reached when people perceive their current activities as relating to future outcomes, so that current events draw meaning from possible future conditions. In fact, most scholars agree that a purpose in life represents a pursuit of some type of aim or goal, but one that it is particularly stable and far-reaching (Damon et al. 2003; Damon 2008).

In this way, purpose serves as a broader motivational aim that influences behavioral patterns and directs short-term goals (McKinght and Kashdan 2009). In particular, a purpose may determine the nature of more proximal strivings (Emmons 1999) and personal projects (Little 2006). As one team of researchers put it, "Purpose is a central, self-organizing life aim that *organizes and stimulates* goals, manages behaviors, and provides a sense of meaning. Purpose *directs* life goals and daily decisions by *guiding* the use of finite resources" (McKnight and Kashdan 2009, p. 242 emphasis added). In many cases, a far-horizon purpose serves as the reason behind more immediate goals and activities. Accordingly, studying hard to get into medical school may represent a worthwhile short-term goal for an individual pursuing a long-term purpose of providing high quality healthcare.

A purposeful aim is one that may never be fully reached, but one that motivates individuals to make progress it. For example, individuals may aspire to reduce homelessness, increase society's appreciation for jazz music, and improve the political climate. While these goals may ever *fully* be achieved, each can imbue an individual's life with an important sense of direction and meaning, and it is the pursuit that matters. This driving aspect of purpose is key to its role as the ultimate motivator. As Ryff and Singer note, "[pursuing one's] life purpose is a dynamic process—the sense that one's life is meaningful and purposeful is an ongoing, day-by-day, constantly unfolding phenomenon, not an end state that is once-and-for-all resolved" (Ryff and Singer 2008, p. 8). Similarly, Emmons notes that ultimate concerns, which are akin to purposes, "represent potentialities rather than actualities in that they are never fully satisfied" (2005, p. 732).

A purpose in life represents a highly motivating commitment. Individuals feel inspired or provoked or compelled by a purpose in life, and consequently, they alter their behavior, align their resources, and direct their efforts to make progress toward their purpose. The goal-directedness inherent in pursuing purpose is underscored by a strong sense of motivation and active engagement in pursuing one's aims.

Finally, the third component of purpose is a sense of personal meaningfulness. Not all of the things we feel motivated to do are particularly meaningful. For instance, an individual may be motivated to lose weight, but this pursuit may not hold long-term, personal significance. A purpose, on the other hand, is central and personally meaningful. For example, Crumbaugh and Maholick (1967) define purpose as "*the ontological significance* of life *from the point of view of the experiencing individual*" (emphasis added, p. 201), and Ryff and Singer (1998) point to the importance of "*feeling that there is meaning* in one's present and past life" (emphasis added, p. 107). Similarly, McKinght and Kashdan (2009) define purpose as a central, self-organizing life aim that organizes and stimulates goals, manages behaviors, and *provides a sense of meaning* (emphasis added, p. 242).

Along with being personally meaningful, purposes tend to be very central to individuals. One conception of purpose refers to this dimension as the "scope" of purpose (McKnight and Kashdan 2009). "Scope refers to how ubiquitous the purpose is in a person's life. A purpose that is central to the person's life and influences all actions, thoughts, and emotions ought to be considered to have a broad scope" (p. 243). So central is the concept of personal meaningfulness that some definitions of purpose equate the construct with meaning (Frankl 1984; Crumbaugh and Maholick 1964, 1968) and others conceive of purpose as a component of meaning (Baumeister 1991; Reker and Wong 1988).

These three elements—commitment, goal-directedness, and personal meaningfulness—are irrefutable components of the construct. They appear in the vast majority of existing definitions of the construct. Like a compass that always points north, a purpose in life consistently orients and motivates an individual toward a personally significant aim. In some conceptions of purpose, these three elements are not only necessary, but they are also considered sufficient for discerning the presence of purpose (Ryff and Singer 1998; Crumbaugh and Maholick 1964; 1967; McKnight and Kashdan 2009).

However, a close reading of Frankl's work suggests there is another component of purpose in addition to these three. That component is a focus on impacting the world beyond-the-self. A life purpose represents a desire to work toward a personally meaningful aim that is not solely self-serving, but that also leads to productive engagement with some aspect of the broader world. According to Frankl a life purpose provides the foundation for human motivation, and he called that motivation "noetic" or,

> the "spiritual" or inspirational and aspirational aspects of the mind. This is not necessarily "religious;" it merely points to a "higher" or non-material side of life. It is another way of saying that "man does not live by bread alone" and that finding a real meaning and purpose in life is not a matter of accumulating "things," but rather of performing some task that causes one to gain some type of feedback, real or imagined, now or in the future, of appreciation, commendation and acceptance from one's fellows (Crumbaugh 1977, p. 901)[1].

Though Crumbaugh and Maholick (1964, 1968) did not emphasize Frankl's beyond-the-self component of purpose in their writing or purpose survey measure, it is clear that Frankl believed the construct included this integral feature. A life purpose represents an aim that is at once personally meaningful and at the same time engages the individual in the broader world. Doing something for one's family, in service of one's God, or on behalf of one's community or country are all ways of being actively engaged in the world beyond-the-self.

The beyond-the-self component of purpose is significant, not only theoretically, but also practically. Empirical research finds that it differentiates people based on important indicators of psychological well-being. Individuals with beyond-the-self aims demonstrate more integrated personality dispositions, improved psychological adjustment, higher levels of achievement, more openness, and greater levels of

[1] Frankl consulted with Crumbaugh and Maholick on this paper, and according to Crumbaugh and Maholick, this definition aligns with Frankl's conception.

life satisfaction than individuals who do not express a commitment to beyond-the-self aims (Bronk and Finch 2010; Mariano and Vaillant 2012). The beyond-the-self conception of purpose is particularly useful from a developmental perspective as it typically is operationalized as a prosocial or noble commitment to an aim beyond the individual.

Interestingly, studies of lay conceptions of purpose reveal that most people consider a purpose in life to include beyond-the-self concerns (Hill et al. 2012). It is also noteworthy that the widely popular *Purpose-Driven Life* (Warren 2002), a book which has sold over 30 million copies and has spawned a cottage industry of purpose-seeking, opens with a simple sentence: "It's not about you" (p. 11). In other words, "it" or the pursuit of purpose, is about something larger than the self.

Finally, the beyond-the-self component of purpose is useful because it helps distinguish *purpose* from the related construct of *meaning*. Many early researchers (Frankl 1984; Ryff and Singer 1998), including Frankl, used the terms interchangeably. However, in the past 10 years, as empirical attention to purpose and meaning has grown, it has become necessary to clearly distinguish these related constructs. Increasingly, it has become accepted that meaning refers to anything that makes one's life seem more significant, while purpose refers to a subset of those sources of meaning that also lead to productive engagement with the world beyond-the-self (Damon 2008; Damon et al. 2003).

Another way purpose and meaning differ has to do with goal orientation. Whereas purpose refers to a personally meaningful, far-horizon aim in life, most conceptions of meaning do not refer to goals or aims. Meaning in life, instead, encompasses both situational meaning and existential meaning (Wong, in press). Situational meaning refers to the way individuals make sense of the world around them, while existential meaning refers to the reason for an individual's existence. Meaning refers to the sense we make out of the world and events around us. It is the way we understand our surroundings and the place we hold relative to them (Parks 2011). Definitions of meaning conceive of the construct as "the sense made of and significance felt regarding the nature of one's being and existence" (Steger et al. 2006, p. 81).

While meaning and purpose are distinct constructs, they are clearly related. The meaning we make of our surroundings helps orient us and allows us to find our place in the world, and the meaning we make of the world around us shapes our sense of self and purpose (Parks 2011). In short, the meaning we find in our existence influences the nature of our purposes.

As a means of encompassing prevailing notions of purpose evident in the literature while at the same time incorporating this critical beyond-the-self component, the following definition of purpose was proposed about 10 years ago: *A purpose in life is a stable and generalized intention that is at once meaningful to the self and at the same time leads to productive engagement with some aspect of the world beyond-the-self* (Damon 2008; Damon et al. 2003). This definition emphasizes the important role of commitment, goal-directedness, and personal meaningfulness along with a focus on beyond-the-self concerns, and as such, it has been widely adopted among researchers studying purpose.

Philosophical Underpinnings

This definition of purpose, like earlier definitions, has been significantly influenced by philosophical conceptions of the construct. Philosophers have long contemplated whether there is a purpose in life, and if so, what it is. Most philosophers agree that lives can feature degrees of purpose or significance and that purpose connotes a "good" that is conceptually distinct from happiness.

Socrates and Plato were certainly interested in the idea of purpose, but likely the most influential early Greek philosopher to contemplate purpose was Aristotle. Aristotle was interested in understanding how people should live and what they should live for. In *Nicomachean Ethics*, (1962) he wrote about the highest good, which he called *eudaimonia*. This Greek term is difficult to translate into English, but it suggests self-actualization, fulfillment, and flourishing. Eudaimonia is a process of living ethically, authentically, and virtuously. It is not a fixed state. Instead, eudaimonia refers to a more stable human thriving that can only be achieved by fulfilling our basic human functions and by performing our characteristic activities. *Eudaimonia* is the result of personally meaningful actions carried out in accordance with virtue and excellence. Aristotle believed that all people possessed particular talents or capacities and we were meant to use those skills to fulfill a particular role, job, or purpose. Working toward that purpose to the best of our ability leads to eudaimonia. The Aristotelian concept of eudaimonia has significantly influenced psychological conceptions of purpose and psychological well-being (Ryff and Keyes 1995; Ryff 1989a, b; Ryff and Singer 2008). See Chap. 3 ("The Role of Purpose in Optimal Human Development") for an elaboration of this point.

In addition to ancient Greek philosophers, more contemporary philosophers have also considered both what the purpose of life is and the function of purpose in human functioning. Purpose theorists often focus on the role of God or other supernatural forces in providing a sense of significance or meaning to one's existence. Most philosophers in this tradition argue that one's existence is more significant to the degree that one fulfills his or her purpose as assigned by God (Metz 2007).

As a philosopher and Protestant theologian, Paul Tillich (1952) was concerned with the notion of faith as ultimate concern. According to Tillich, philosophy poses the ontological question, *what is the meaning of the human experience*, and theology offers the answer, *faith*. Leading a life that demonstrates one's commitment to God is the solution to the ontological threat of non-being; accordingly, faith imbues life with purpose. Individuals must "participate meaningfully in their original creations" (p. 46) in order to encounter the meaning required to stave off the extreme anxiety associated with non-being, or meaninglessness. "The anxiety of meaninglessness is anxiety about the loss of an ultimate concern, of the meaning which gives meaning to all meanings" (p. 47). In this view, one's ultimate concern, or purpose, frames all other personally meaningful aims.

Similarly, another more contemporary philosopher, Robert Nozick (1981), saw the search for "ultimate" purpose or meaning as God-centered. However, Nozick did not view God as the ultimate source of purpose, but instead as the ultimate source of infinity. Meaning in a finite life, he argued, could only be derived from another condition that has meaning (Cooper 2005; Nozick 1981). For example, an individual might find meaning through his or her offspring, and that offspring might derive meaning through his or her work, and so on. In this way, individuals can find meaning through their relations with others or their activities, but those sources of meaning must likewise derive meaning from yet another source. This chain of relationships must end at some point, and meaning can only be found through a connection with something so all-encompassing that it cannot find meaning beyond itself. This "something" is God. In this way, consistent with the proposed definition of purpose, Nozick notes that purpose in life transcends the limits of the self (Nozick 1981, 1989).

In addition to philosophers' beyond-the-self assumptions about purpose, it is also interesting to note the central role of God and faith in these philosophies of purpose. Consistent with this, the majority of the psychological research on different types of purpose has focused on religious-oriented aims, as opposed to service, familial, or career-oriented purposes. A full discussion of religious and other types of purposes can be found in Chap. 7, ("The Experience of Purpose among Diverse Groups").

Of course, there are many other philosophers who have contemplated life purposes, both directly and indirectly, and many who have focused on more secular approaches to finding purpose (e.g. Albert Camus and Jean-Paul Sartre), but the preceding discussion addresses some of the philosophies that have had the greatest influence on psychological writings on the topic. As such, while the preceding brief discussion is by no means meant to be exhaustive, it offers a useful starting point for considering the philosophical foundations of the purpose in life construct.

Purpose in Theories of Optimal Development

The preceding philosophies have influenced not only our understanding of what purpose is, but also the way we view purpose in relation to optimal human functioning. In the past 20 years, a sea change has swept through the study and practice of psychology. Whereas psychologists used to focus on ways of reducing suffering, shortcomings, and other afflictions of the human condition, we now recognize this aim as too narrow. We need to do more. Specifically, we need to gain a deeper understanding of how all people can lead fuller, more connected, more productive, and more meaningful lives.

This new positive psychology paradigm has led to research on a wide range of constructs that support optimal human development (Seligman 2011; Seligman and Csikszentmihalyi 2000). In conjunction with this movement, developmental psychologists interested in promoting healthy development among young people have focused on understanding ways of expanding and supporting positive youth development (Benson 2006; Bundick et al. 2010; Damon 2004; Lerner 2004). Optimal growth, among adults and young people, is not characterized merely by the absence of problems, such as drug abuse and antisocial behavior, but also by the presence of adaptive characteristics and capacities.

So what exactly constitutes optimal human functioning? Sitting around a conference table at the Stanford Center on Adolescence 12 years ago, my colleagues and I contemplated this question. Interested in devising a measure of positive youth development, we wondered what should we include? What are the components of positive human development? What are its indicators? What are its outcomes? Though debate still exists around these questions, researchers have developed several useful theories of positive human development, and pursuing a purpose in life is a core component of each of them.

Early in the study of positive psychology, rather than focusing directly on ways that people thrive and flourish, researchers focused on ways individuals effectively coped with difficult circumstances and other hardships. Accordingly, early theories focused on constructs such as resiliency (Werner and Smith 1992) and hardiness (Kobasa 1979). Both are personality characteristics evident in individuals who successfully cope with challenging obstacles. Resiliency is manifest through having a sense of purpose and a belief in a bright future (Benard 1991), whereas hardiness is evident among individuals who demonstrate a sense of challenge (the belief that life is ever changing and that these changes are opportunities for growth), control (the belief that individuals can influence events around them), and commitment (the belief that it is worthwhile to become deeply involved in what one does; Kobasa 1979). Commitment is a central component of both purpose and hardiness, and individuals who display commitment tend to demonstrate vigorous involvement in their lives. Rather than being passive by-standers, committed individuals actively insert themselves into the important activities in their lives. Individuals cannot sustain a purpose in life without making a commitment to a particular aim, and hardy individuals who demonstrate commitment tend to be well equipped to cope with challenges. In this way, purpose, hardiness, and healthy human development are all related.

Other early models of well-being similarly focused on an individual's ability to bounce back from hardship. For example, Aaron Antonovky (1987) proposed a theory of salutogenesis, in which rather than focusing on illness or challenges, individuals focus on resources available to help them overcome difficult circumstances. Antonovky (1987) was interested in understanding how it was that individuals could survive traumatic events, such as the death of a loved one or spending time in deprived environments, and emerge psychologically unscarred. Individuals who not only survive, but thrive, he argued, have a strong sense of coherence in their lives. Coherence represents a global orientation that expresses the extent to which one has a pervasive and enduring feeling of confidence that (1) stimuli deriving from one's internal and external environments in the course of living are structured, predictable, and explicable; (2) resources are available to help meet the demands posed by these stimuli; and (3) demands are challenges, worthy of investment and engagement. In other words, a sense of coherence consists of comprehensibility (the extent to which life generally seem to make sense), manageability (the extent to which individuals perceive they have the resources required to handle challenges), and meaningfulness (the extent to which people believe their lives are worthy and important). The meaningfulness component of this model overlaps significantly with purpose. Individuals who believe their lives are meaningful are likely to report their lives have a purpose. Based on this model, feeling that life is meaningful or purposeful is an important element of effective coping.

Theories of hardiness, resiliency, and coherence reveal different ways in which purpose figures into well-being. These and other early positive psychology constructs focus on the ability to cope effectively and endure hardship. As such, each of these models starts from a position of struggle or adversity. Rather than assuming negative starting points, more contemporary theories of positive psychology focus on identifying ways in which all people, regardless of where they start, can be well and thrive.

Carol Ryff and Burton Singer's (1988) theory of psychological well-being provides a useful example of this. Their theory of eudaimonia, based on Aristotle's philosophy, suggests that holding a positive opinion of oneself (self-acceptance), being able to choose or create contexts appropriate for one's psychological condition (environmental mastery), having warm and trusting relationships and being able to love (positive relations), continually developing one's potential (personal growth), being self-determined and independent (autonomy), and having goals, aspirations, and direction in life (purpose) all converge to predict psychological well-being (Ryff and Singer 2008). Having a purpose in life, or a sense that one is moving in a personally meaningful direction, represents one of six components of psychological well-being. Collectively the presence of these six factors, predicts positive functioning (e.g. life satisfaction and psychological health) and is inversely related to negative functioning (e.g. depression and anxiety; Ryff and Singer 1996). However these six factors do not contribute equally to well-being; purpose has been found to be one of the most important contributors to positive mental health (Ryff and Singer 2008). High purpose scores are also associated with important markers of biological health (Boyle et al. 2010; Ryff and Keyes 1995; Ryff and Singer 2002; Ryff et al. 2004). The consistent relationship between purpose and both psychological and physical well-being demonstrated by this model underscores the importance of purpose, not only in models of coping, but also in influential models of thriving.

Many other more recent positive psychology theories similarly consider purpose to be a critical component of optimal human functioning. For example, Seligman's (2002) theory of authentic happiness identifies three key elements of optimal development, including positive emotion, engagement, and meaning. Experiencing each of these components is likely to produce a sense of satisfaction with one's life, but according to Seligman, they lead to qualitatively different types of life satisfaction. Positive emotions are required for a pleasant life. We all seek to do things, like get a massage or eat an ice cream sundae, that make us feel good for a while. In short, leading a pleasant life is a useful path to temporary contentment. Next, engagement, similar to flow (Csikszentmihalyi 1997), represents another way of achieving satisfaction. By being engaged and experiencing flow, which we can do by playing music, running, painting, or writing, etc., we lose ourselves in the activities we love. When we participate in activities that are simultaneously challenging and enjoyable, we experience flow, but again the positive feelings associated with this experience are relatively short lived. When we move on to other activities, they fade. Positive emotions and engagement lead to brief states of contentment. To experience enduring satisfaction or well-being, people need to seek meaning and purpose for their lives. According to Seligman, having a sense of purpose, or a sense of belonging to or working toward something bigger than the self, represents the third and most enduring element of authentic happiness.

Over the years, Seligman's thinking on optimal human development has evolved. In 2011 he published a book that proposed a revised theory of optimal human development, which conceptualizes flourishing, as opposed to life satisfaction, as the ultimate aim of optimal human development. Whereas life satisfaction is disproportionately influenced by our fleeting moods, well-being is a the result of a constellation of elements. The primary contributors to flourishing include positive emotion, engagement, positive relationships, accomplishments, and—again—purpose in life (Seligman 2011).

A related model of optimal development emphasizes the importance of character strengths and virtues in psychological well-being (Peterson and Seligman 2004). The Values in Action (VIA) classification provides a useful framework for identifying and better understanding strengths of character. According to the VIA classification, there are six primary strengths of character, including courage, love, justice, temperance, wisdom, and transcendence. These six broad categories each encompass a group of 24 specific virtues. However, factor analysis using the VIA reveals only four factors, including temperance strengths (e.g. prudence and self-regulation); intellectual strengths (e.g. love of learning, curiosity); other-oriented strengths (e.g. kindness and teamwork); and transcendent strengths (e.g. gratitude and purpose in life) (Park and Peterson 2006). Transcendent strengths of character, which encompass purpose, are hypothesized to enhance development by providing individuals with a sense of direction and connection to others (Gillham et al. 2011). The VIA classification model is designed to make it easier to identify thriving individuals and programs that promote healthy development (Peterson and Seligman 2004). It is interesting to note, though, that in this model as in the other models of positive health, purpose holds a central role.

While the preceding theories address adult well-being, a parallel body of research addresses positive youth development. The Search Institute's developmental assets approach is based on a leading theory of positive youth development. According to Peter Benson, the late President and CEO of the Search Institute, developmental assets support healthy growth among young people (Benson 2006). Developmental assets include critical dispositions, relationships, and opportunities that can be fostered at home, at school, and in communities. Assets form the building blocks of healthy development, and the more assets an individual possesses, the more likely that individual is to thrive. Assets are divided into two groups: external and internal assets. The 20 external assets focus on the nature and quality of the young person's environment. They include external support (e.g. family support, caring community), empowerment (e.g. communities value youth and view them as resources), appropriate boundaries and expectations (e.g. positive peer influence, family has clear rules), and constructive use of time (e.g. creative activities, religious community). The 20 internal assets highlight capacities that should be fostered in youth, including a commitment to learning (e.g. achievement motivation, school engagement), positive values (e.g. caring, responsibility), social competencies (e.g. cultural competence, peaceful conflict resolution), and positive identity. Included in positive identity is a sense of purpose, which serves to provide "young people a base for direction and meaning" (p. 56). In this conception of positive youth development, purpose is simultaneously a key component and indicator of young people's well-being.

Benson's conception of optimal youth development emphasizes the dynamic interplay between the healthy growth of young people and supportive communities. Rich Lerner and colleagues (Lerner et al. 2003) similarly conceive of positive youth development in context. Young people, they argue, are resources that communities should invest in and support (Lerner 2003). Consequently, Lerner and his colleagues have posited a developmental systems model of healthy human development in which an other-oriented purpose represents the outcome of healthy development. According to this team of researchers, positive youth development involves flexibility and adaptive regulation of the person-context relationship. In short, communities should support the healthy development of youth in order to produce a population of individuals with a vested interest in promoting the health of their communities. Exactly what constitutes healthy development is highly influenced by society, culture, and time, but in the United States and other Westernized cultures individual freedom, equity, and democracy are highly valued, and these values are reflected in Lerner's (2004) Five C's of healthy development: competence, confidence, character, social connection, and caring or compassion. These attributes are regarded as healthy outcomes of functionally adaptive developmental regulations. To the extent that adolescents demonstrate these five characteristics, they can be said to be thriving. Young people who demonstrate the 5 C's are also likely to enact a sixth C, contribution (Lerner 2004; Lerner et al. 2005). Contributing means acting in ways that benefit the broader world. Accordingly, in this view, individuals who demonstrate the 5C's, are also likely to demonstrate signs of purpose.

From models of resiliency to theories of thriving, purpose holds a central position in varied conceptions of optimal human functioning. While other elements appear in some models of well-being but not others, purpose appears in each of these leading theories. The role of purpose varies by theory (e.g. in some it is a contributor to well-being, in others an outcome, etc), but what is clear is that purpose is an important component of optimal human development.

The Nature of Purpose

While it is clear that purpose is central to healthy growth, preceding discussions of purpose tend to assume that the construct is exclusively positive, moral, or noble in nature, and based on the proposed definition, this need not be the case. The primary components of purpose—commitment, goal-directedness, personal meaningfulness, and a beyond-the-self focus—are not inherently positive. Just as forms of engagement in the broader world can be noble or ignoble, moral or immoral, so too can a purpose be positive or negative. For example, Hitler presumably found purpose in his attempts to rid the world of Jews, just as Mother Teresa likely found purpose in her work ministering to the impoverished and ill. In both instances these individuals were engaged in the broader world, working toward personally meaningful aims. While ignoble purposes are not excluded based on this definition, most contemporary studies focus on noble or at least neutral aims. Accordingly, most of the research presented in this book assumes a positive or at least neutral manifestation of purpose.

Some may argue that distinguishing between moral and immoral purposes is impossible, but it is not. The interested reader is directed to *Youth Purpose: Conclusions from a Working Conference of Leading Scholars* (Bronk et al. 2004) for a fuller explanation of how such a distinction can be drawn. In general, however, it is important to keep in mind that for a purpose to be considered noble "the *why* of the deed as well as its *how* must be guided by a strong moral sense" (Damon 2003, p. 12).

Beyond the nature of purpose, it is also interesting to consider the number of purposes one is likely to be inspired by. Based on the definition, a person may have more than one purpose in life. However, in practice, purposes tend to be closely related to one another as individuals have only so much time, energy, and effort to allocate to any particular aspiration (Damon 2008). A recent study of youth purpose exemplars featured a young woman who wanted to serve God by providing medical care to people in need (Bronk 2012). While this young woman was guided by two purposes (service to God and service to the needy), far from being at odds with one another, her aspirations represented overlapping aims. These kinds of related purposes are typical not only among exemplars, but also among youth with less highly developed but perhaps more common forms of purpose (Bronk and Finch 2010). This book will review these studies of purpose and others.

Scope and Outline of the Book

Scientific research on purpose was virtually non-existent before the 1960s, and until roughly the past 10 years, it has continued to be rare. However, along with the launch of the positive psychology movement, the number of empirical studies on purpose has increased substantially. This book attempts to review and synthesize the rapidly growing body of theoretical and empirical research available on the construct. In particular, this book focuses on the historical, landmark studies of purpose and on more recent empirical studies on the topic. It also focuses primarily on studies of purpose as opposed to studies of meaning or other related constructs. However at times, especially when research on purpose is unavailable, findings from studies of closely related concepts, especially meaning, ultimate concerns, aspirations, wisdom, generativity, and fidelity, are addressed to shed light on as of yet unexamined aspects of purpose.

It is also important to note that purpose is largely an adolescent and emerging adulthood phenomenon. Its development is closely tied to the development of identity (Bronk 2011; Damon 2008; Erikson 1968; 1980), a topic that will be discussed more fully in Chap. 4 ("Purpose Across the Lifespan"). Adolescents, unlike younger children, are cognitively capable of considering existential questions, such as: What is worthwhile in my life? What do I particularly care about? What do I hope to accomplish? And, tied up in these kinds of questions is a search for the ultimate purpose in life. In this way, the search for purpose is based on the self-understanding and self-knowledge that typically emerges during the second decade of life. Not only are most adolescents cognitively and emotionally ready to explore issues of personal meaningfulness, but they are also ready to consider their aspirations in the context of their future plans as they reflect on ways that they can apply their talents to fill personally meaningful social needs (Damon 2008; Fry 1998). Purpose becomes salient to adolescents as they consider who they are and what they hope to accomplish in their lives. The commitments young people make often set them on a trajectory that endures into adulthood. Consequently, while this book offers an overview of the purpose construct from a lifespan perspective, the bulk of the research presented focuses on purpose during the adolescent and emerging adult life stages.

Being able to measure the purpose construct accurately and efficiently is key to increasing our understanding of the construct. Accordingly, the second chapter of this book discusses the surveys, interviews, diary reviews, and document review approaches that have been utilized to study the purpose construct. Each of these methods has strengths and weaknesses that are also addressed in this chapter. When relevant, subsequent discussions reference the measures used in the studies for which findings are reported.

Purpose is a relevant topic primarily because of its central role in optimal human functioning. To date, multiple studies have concluded that purpose supports psychological well-being, and the construct is increasingly associated with improved physical health as well. In addition to identifying health outcomes that correlate with purpose, Chap. 3 also synthesizes research that illuminates the mechanism through which purpose promotes healthy development.

Next, purpose is a developmental construct. While it represents a healthy component of development at all stages in the lifespan, its role and prevalence varies based on age. As already noted, the development of purpose is closely tied to the development of identity. The symbiotic relationship between these important constructs is one focus of Chap. 4. This chapter also synthesizes theoretical and empirical research relevant to the developmental trajectory of purpose.

Chapter 5 focuses on the ways purposes develop and are supported over time. It features a discussion of the potential evolutionary roots and the developmental origins of purpose. The role parents, peers, mentors, and communities can play in fostering purpose among young people is also addressed, and a handful of intervention studies, which suggest ways purpose can be nurtured, are reviewed.

Inspiring purposes in life are often discovered in religious, career, family, and service-oriented activities. Chapter 6 summarizes empirical research on these different types of purpose. In addition to outlining the challenges associated with categorizing purposes, this chapter also addresses the way different kinds of purposes develop, are supported, and contribute to well-being.

The experience of leading a life of purpose is the topic of Chap. 7. More specifically, this chapter features research on the daily and longer-term experience of leading a life of purpose among diverse groups, including urban, suburban, and rural youth as well as high ability and more typical youth and individuals from different ethnic backgrounds.

For a full understanding of any developmental construct, including purpose, research is needed not only on deficient and typical forms, but also on exemplary or highly developed forms of the construct. Chapter 8 outlines the parameters of the exemplar methodology and explains why this emerging methodology is an important tool for understanding developmental constructs, such as purpose. This chapter also highlights findings from a longitudinal study of youth purpose exemplars. The development of purpose, its relation to identity development, and the mechanism behind the association between purpose and positive youth development are discussed.

Finally, after spending years conducting research on purpose and reviewing the growing literature on the construct, it is clear that much has been gleaned from well-crafted, empirical studies. Additionally, theoretical research sheds important light on other important aspects of the purpose construct. However, while existing research provides a strong foundation for our growing understanding of the construct, it is just that, a foundation. More work is needed, and the final chapter of this book highlights gaps in the literature and identifies future directions for research on the purpose in life construct.

References

Antonovsky, A. (1987). *Unraveling the mystery of health*. San Francisco: Jossey Bass.

Aristotle. (1962). *Nicomachean Ethics. Translated by Martin Ostwald*. Indianapolis: The Library of Liberal Arts.

Baumeister, R. (1991). *Meanings of life*. New York: The Guilford Press.

Benard, B. (1991). *Fostering resiliency in kids: Protective factors in the family, school, and community*. San Francisco: Far West Laboratory for Educational Research and Development.

Benson, P. L. (2006). *All kids are our kids: What communities must do to raise caring and responsible children and adolescents* (2nd ed.). San Francisco: Jossey Bass.

Boyd, B. (2009). Purpose-driven life. *American Scholar, 78*(2), 24–34.

Boyle, P. A., Buchman, A. S., Barnes, L. L., James, B. D., & Bennett, D. A. (2010). Association between life space and risk of mortality in advanced age. *Journal of the American Geriatrics Society, 58*(10), 1925–1930.

Bronk, K. C. (2011). Portraits of purpose: The role of purpose in identity formation. *A special issue on Instructing for and Supporting Youth Purpose in New Directions in Youth Development, 132,* 31–44.

Bronk, K. C. (2012). A grounded theory of youth purpose. *Journal of Adolescent Research, 27,* 78–109. http://dx.doi.org/10.1177/0743558411412958.

Bronk, K. C., & Finch, W. H. (2010). Adolescent characteristics by type of long-term aim in life. *Applied Developmental Science, 14*(1), 1–10.

Bronk, K. C., Menon, J. L., & Damon, W. (2004). *Youth purpose: Conclusions from a working conference of leading scholars*. West Conshohocken: John Templeton Foundation Press.

Bundick, M. J., Yeager, D. S., King, P. E., & Damon, W. (2010). Thriving across the lifespan. In R. M. Lerner, M. E. Lamb, A. M. Freund, & W. F. Overton (Eds.), *Handbook of life-span development, vol. 1: Cognition, biology and methods* (pp. 882–923). Hoboken: Wiley.

Cooper, D. (2005). Life and meaning. *Ratio, 18,* 125–137.

Crumbaugh, J. C. (1968). Cross-validation of Purpose in Life Test based on Frankl's concepts. *Journal of Individual Psychology, 24,* 74–81.

Crumbaugh, J. C. (1971). Frankl's logotherapy: A new orientation to counseling. *Journal of Religion and Health, 10,* 373–386.

Crumbaugh, J. C. (1977). *Manual of instructions for the Seeking of Noetic Goals test.* Munster: Psychometric Affiliates.

Crumbaugh, J. C. & Henrion R. (2001). How to find meaning and purpose in life for the third millennium. *The International Forum for Logotherapy, 24*(1), 1–9.

Crumbaugh, J. C., & Maholick, L. T. (1964). An experimental study in existentialism: The psychometric approach to Frankl's concept of noogenic neurosis. *Journal of Clinical Psychology, 20,* 589–596.

Crumbaugh, J. C., & Maholick, L. T. (1967). *An experimental study in existentialism: The psychometric approach to Frankl's concept of Noogenic Neurosis. Psychotherapy and existentialism* (pp. 183–197). New York: Washington Square Press.

Csikszentmihalyi, M. (1997). *Finding flow: The psychology of engagement with everyday life.* New York: Basic Books.

Damon, W. (2003). *Noble purpose: The joy of living a meaningful life*. Radnor: Templeton Foundation Press.

Damon, W. (2004). What is positive youth development? *Annals of the American Academy of Political and Social Science, 591,* 13–23.

Damon, W. (2008). *The path to purpose: How young people find their calling in life*. New York: The Free Press.

Damon, W., Menon, J., & Bronk, K. C. (2003). The development of purpose during adolescence. *Applied Developmental Science, 7*(3), 119–128.

van Deurzen-Smith, E. (1997). *Everyday mysteries: Existential dimensions of psychotherapy*. New York: Routledge.

Emmons, R. A. (1999). *The psychology of ultimate concerns: Motivation and spirituality in personality*. New York: Guilford Press.

Emmons, R. A. (2005). Striving for the sacred: Personal goals, life meaning, and religion. *Journal of Social Issues, 61*(4), 731–745.

Erikson, E. H. (1968). *Identity youth and crisis*. New York: W.W. Norton & Company Inc.

Erikson, E. H. (1980). *Identity and the life cycle (paperback)*. New York: W.W. Norton & Company Inc.

Fabry, J. (1988). *Guideposts to meaning: Discovering what really matters*. Oakland: Harbinger Publications.

Frankl, V. E. (1959). *Man's search for meaning: An introduction to logotherapy.* Boston: Beacon Press.

Frankl, V. E. (1979). *The unheard cry for meaning: Psychotherapy and humanism*. New York: Touchstone.

Frankl, V. E. (1984). *Man's search for meaning: An introduction to logotherapy, revised and updated*. Boston: Beacon Press.

Fry, P. S. (1998). The development of personal meaning and wisdom in adolescence: A reexamination of moderating and consolidating factors an influences. In P. T. P. Wong (Ed.), *The human quest for meaning: A handbook of psychological research and clinical application* (2nd ed., (pp. 91–110). New York: Routledge.

Gillham, J., Adams-Deutsch, Z., Werner, J., Rievich, K., Coulter-Heindl, V., Linkins, M., Winder, B., Peterson, C., Park, N., Abenavoli, R., Contero, A., & Seligman, M. E. P. (2011). Character strengths predict subjective well-being during adolescence. *The Journal of Positive Psychology, 6*(1), 31–44.

Hill, P. L., Burrow, A., O'Dell, A. C., & Thornton, M. A. (2012). Classifying adolescents' conceptions of purpose in life. *Journal of Positive Psychology, 5*(6), 466–473.

Klinger, E. (1998). The search for meaning in evolutionary perspective. In P. T. P. Wong & P. S. Fry (Eds.), *The human quest for meaning* (pp. 27–50). Mahwah: Lawrence Erlbaum Associates.

Kobasa, S. C. (1979). Stressful life events, personality, and health. *Journal of Personality and Social Psychology, 37,* 1–11.

Korotkov, D. (1998). The sense of coherence: Making sense out of chaos. In P. T. P. Wong & P. S. Fry (Eds.), *The human quest for meaning* (pp. 51–70). Mahwah: Lawrence Erlbaum Associates.

Lerner, R. M. (2003). Developmental assets and asset building communities: A view of the issues. In R. M. Lerner & P. L. Benson (Eds.), *Developmental assets and asset-building communities: Implications for research, policy, and practice*. New York: Kluwer Academic, Plenum Publishers.

Lerner, R. (2004). *Liberty: Thriving and civic engagement among America's youth.* Thousand Oaks: Sage Publications.

Lerner, R. M., Dowling, E. M., & Anderson, P. M. (2003). Positive youth development: Thriving as the basis of personhood and civil society. *Applied Developmental Science, 7*(3), 172–180.

Lerner, R. M., Lerner, J. V., Almerigi, J. B., Theokas, C., Phelps, E., Getsdottir, S., Naudeau, S., Leicic, H., Alberts, A., Ma, L., Smith, L. M., Bobek, D. L., Richman-Raphael, D., & Simpson, I. (2005). Positive youth development, participation in community youth development programs, and community contributions of fifth-grade adolescents: Findings from the first wave of the 4-H study of positive youth development. *Journal of Early Adolescence, 25*(1), 17–71. doi:10.1177/0272431604272461.

Little, B. R. (2006). *Personal project pursuit: Goals, action, and human functioning.* New York: Lawrence Erlbaum Associates.

Maddi, S. R. (1998). Creating meaning through making decisions. In P. T. P. Wong & P. S. Fry (Eds.), *The human quest for meaning* (pp. 3–26). Mahwah: Lawrence Erlbaum Associates.

Mariano, J. M., & Vaillant, G. (2012). Youth purpose among the 'Greatest Generation.' *Journal of Positive Psychology*. doi:10.1080/17439760.2012.686624.

McKnight, P. E., & Kashdan, T. B. (2009). Purpose in life as a system that creates and sustains health and well-being: An integrative, testable theory. *Review of General Psychology, 13*(3), 242–251.

Melton, A. M. A., Schulenberg, S. E. (2008). On the measurement of meaning: Logotherapy's empirical contributions to humanist psychology. *The Humanist Psychologist, 36,* 31–44.

Metz, T. (2007). The meaning of life. *Stanford encyclopedia of philosophy*. Stanford: Metaphysics Research Lab, CSLI. http://plato.stanford.edu/entries/life-meaning/. Accessed 13 May 2011.

Nozick, R. (1981). *Philosophical explanations*. Cambridge: Harvard University Press.

Nozick, R. (1989). *The examined life*. New York: Simon & Schuster.

Park, N., & Peterson, C. (2006). Moral competence and character strengths among adolescents: The development and validation of the values in action inventory of strengths for youth. *Journal of Adolescence, 29,* 891–909.

Parks, S. D. (2011). *Big questions, worthy dreams: Mentoring emerging adults in their search for meaning, purpose, and faith* (Revised 10th anniversary ed.). San Francisco: Jossey Bass.

Peterson, C., & Seligman, M. E. P. (2004). *Character strengths and virtues: A handbook and classification.* New York: Oxford University Press; Washington DC: American Psychological Association.

Reker, G. T., & Wong, P. T. P. (1988). Towards a theory of personal meaning. In J. E. Birren & V. L. Bengston (Eds.), *Emergent theories of aging* (pp. 214–246). New York: Springer.

Ryff, C. D. (1989a). Beyond Ponce de Leon and life satisfaction: New directions in the quest for successful aging. *International Journal of Behavioral Development, 12,* 35–55.

Ryff, C. D. (1989b). Happiness is everything, or is it? Explorations on the meaning of psychological well-being. *Journal of Personality and Social Psychology, 57,* 1069–1081.

Ryff, C. D., & Keyes, C. L. (1995). The structure of psychological well-being revisited. *Journal of Personality and Social Psychology, 69*(4), 719–727.

Ryff, C. D., & Singer, B. (1996). Psychological well-being: Meaning, measurement, and implications for psychotherapy research. *Psychotherapy and Psychosomatics, 65,* 14–23.

Ryff, C. D., & Singer, B. H. (1998). The contours of positive human health. *Psychological Inquiry, 19,* 1–28.

Ryff, C. D., & Singer, B. H. (2002). From social structure to biology: Integrative science in pursuit of human health and well-being. In C. R. Snyder & S. J. Lopez (Eds.), *Handbook of positive psychology* (pp. 541–554). Oxford: University Press.

Ryff, C. D., & Singer, B. H. (2008). Know thyself and become what you are: A eudaimonic approach to psychological well-being. *Journal of Happiness Studies, 9,* 13–39.

Ryff, C. D., Singer, B., & Love, G. D. (2004). Positive health: Connecting well-being with biology. *Philosophical Transactions Royal Society London B, Biological Sciences, 359,* 1383–1394. doi:10.1098/rstb.2004.1521.

Schulenberg, S. (2004). A psychometric investigation of logotherapy measures and the Outcome Questionnaire (OQ-45.2). *North American Journal of Psychology, 6*(3), 477–92.

Seligman, M. E. P. (2002). *Authentic happiness: Using the new positive psychology to realize your potential for lasting fulfillment.* New York: Free Press.

Seligman, M. E. P. (2011). *Flourish: A visionary new understanding of happiness and well-being.* New York: Free Press.

Seligman, M. E. P., & Csikszentmihalyi, M. (2000). Positive psychology: An introduction. *American Psychologist, 55,* 5–14.

Sheldon, K. M., & King, L. A. (2001). *Why positive psychology is necessary. American Psychologist, 56,* 216–217.

Steger, M. F., Frazier, P., Oishi, S., & Kaler, M. (2006). The meaning in life questionnaire: Assessing the presence of and search for meaning in life. *Journal of Counseling Psychology, 53*(1), 80–91.

Tillich, P. (1952). *The courage to be*. New Haven: Yale University Press.

Van Dyke, C. J., & Elias, M. J. (2007). How forgiveness, purpose, and religiosity are related to the mental health and well-being of youth: A review of the literature. *Mental Health, Religion, & Culture, 10*(4), 395–415.

Warren, R. (2002). *The purpose-driven life: What on earth am I here for?* Grand Rapids: Zondervan.

Werner, E., & Smith, R. (1992). *Overcoming the odds: High-risk children from birth to adulthood.* New York: Cornell University Press.

Wong, P. T. P. (in press). The positive psychology of meaning in life and well-being. In A. C. Michalos (Ed.), *Encyclopedia of quality of life research.* Boston: Springer.

Yalom, I. D. (1980). Existential psychotherapy. New York: Basic Books.

Chapter 2
Measuring Purpose

Given the multiple dimensions and subjective nature of the purpose in life construct, measuring it presents a challenge (Melton and Schulenberg 2008). Perhaps because of that, a range of methodological approaches has been used to study purpose. Surveys, interviews, rankings, diary studies, and historical document reviews have been utilized to assess purpose and related constructs. Additionally, measures have been created for use with adolescent, emerging adult, and adult samples.

In line with the history of psychological research, early measures of purpose focused on assessing areas of deficit (Melton and Schulenberg 2008). Tools were developed to study purposelessness among individuals who were depressed, addicted to drugs or alcohol, or otherwise psychologically unfit (e.g. Crumbaugh 1968; Crumbaugh and Maholick 1964; Reker 1977). However, in conjunction with the growth of positive psychological research, more recent assessments of purpose tend to be growth-oriented (e.g. Bronk 2008, 2011, 2012; Bronk et al. 2009, 2010; Damon 2008). Rather than emphasizing the lack of purpose, these studies focus on the positive correlates of leading a life of purpose.

Following is an overview of the tools most commonly used to measure purpose from both deficit and growth-oriented perspectives. The following discussion features measurement tools that have been used with some regularity in empirical studies and that were designed to assess a conception of purpose similar to one put forth in this book.

Surveys Aligned with Frankl's Conception of Purpose

Surveys are the most common assessment tool for the study of purpose, and Viktor Frankl (1959) developed the first psychological survey of purpose in life. Called the Frankl Questionnaire, this self-report measure consists of a relatively informal set of 13 questions. It was created to both assess Frankl's Will to Meaning assumption and to evaluate the degree of purpose present among his patients. He believed that when individuals were unable to find a purpose for their lives they suffered varying degrees of existential frustration, typically manifest as boredom, apathy, or

K. C. Bronk, *Purpose in Life*, DOI 10.1007/978-94-007-7491-9_2,

depression. According to Frankl approximately 20 % of patients seeking psychological counseling suffer from a severe lack of purpose in life (noogenic neurosis) and 55 % of the general public suffers from at least some degree of purposelessness (existential vacuum) (Crumbaugh and Maholick 1964; Crumbaugh 1968). Frankl's evaluation of the presence of purpose depended largely on an individual's response to one questionnaire item, "Do you feel your life is without purpose?" (Crumbaugh and Maholick 1964). Participant responses are coded from "1: no or very low level of purpose or meaning" to "3: high purpose in life present" and are added to scores on the other 12 questions to determine the individual's purpose level.

Frankl used his measure for clinical rather than research purposes. However, two individuals used the measure to conduct empirical studies. Crumbaugh and Maholick (1964) administered the Frankl Questionnaire to a population of psychiatric and more typical adults and found more typical individuals consistently scored higher on purpose than psychiatric patients did, supporting Frankl's theory about the relationship between purpose and mental health. However, given that the measure's reliability and validity have not been assessed, researchers (Reker 1977) have called into question the adequacy of the Frankl Questionnaire as an independent measure of purpose.

Crumbaugh and Maholick agreed that the Frankl Questionnaire was limited as a research tool, so they created a new survey of purpose designed to apply "the principles of existential philosophy to clinical practice" (1964, p. 200). The idea that mental illness could result from existential factors, such as a lack of purpose, went against conventional wisdom at the time (Damon et al. 2003; Kotchen 1960). Behaviorism and psychoanalytical theories prevailed, but Crumbaugh and Maholick, were eager to further test Frankl's controversial thesis.

In consultation with Frankl, Crumbaugh and Maholick (1964) developed the most widely used measure of purpose to date (Pinquart 2002). Their Purpose in Life Test (PIL) improves upon the Frankl Questionnaire, and as such it relies on Frankl's conception of purpose, or "the ontological significance of life from the point of view of the experiencing individual" (Crumbaugh and Maholick 1964, p. 201), and tests Frankl's Will to Meaning assumption (Crumbaugh and Maholick 1964, 1981). In particular, the survey assesses the degree to which individuals strive to make meaning of their conscious experiences and the degree to which that meaning leaves individuals feeling as though their lives are worthwhile and significant (Crumbaugh and Henrion 2001). However, it does not assess an individual's commitment to issues beyond-the-self (Damon et al. 2003).

The PIL consists of three parts: parts A, B, and C. Since only part A is objectively scored, it is the only part that is regularly used in empirical studies of purpose. Part B asks participants to complete 13 sentences about purpose and Part C asks them to compose a paragraph about their personal aspirations. Part A originally consisted of 25-items, but following pilot tests about half of the items were discarded or revised and new questions were added. A 22-item measure resulted (Crumbaugh and Maholick 1964). For simplicity sake, two-reverse scored items are typically omitted in empirical studies using the PIL, leaving a 20-item measure (Crumbaugh 1968; Crumbaugh and Maholick 1981). This 20-item version of the PIL is a self-report measure of attitudes and beliefs that includes statements such as, "I am usually," with response options that range from "1: completely bored" to "7: exuberant, enthusiastic," and "In life I have, 1: no goals or aims at all—7: very clear goals and aims." The total scale score is obtained by summing item scores. Raw scores of 113 and above are typically interpreted as high purpose, scores of 92–112 reflect moderate levels of purpose, and scores of 92 and below suggest a lack of life purpose (Crumbaugh and Maholick 1964). As expected, the PIL and the Frankl Questionnaire are positively correlated ($r = .68$; $p < .05$) (Crumbaugh and Maholick 1967).

The PIL has been administered to a wide range of individuals including women in Junior League (Crumbaugh and Maholick 1964), college students (Crumbaugh 1968; Crumbaugh and Maholick 1964), hospitalized individuals (Crumbaugh 1968), people suffering from alcoholism (Crumbaugh and Maholick 1964; Crumbaugh 1968), psychiatric patients (Crumbaugh and Maholick 1964), business professionals (Bonebright et al. 2000; Crumbaugh 1968), members of religious groups (Crumbaugh 1968), and inmates (Reker 1977). Modified versions of the PIL have also been administered to geriatric (Hutzell 1995), adult (Reker and Peacock 1981), and adolescent populations (Hutzell and Finck 1994; Jeffries 1995). The measure has been translated into a variety of languages, including Chinese (C-PIL; Shek 1993; Shek et al. 1987), Japanese (J-PIL; Okado 1998) and Swedish (Jonsen et al. 2010).

PIL scores correlate with many measures of psychological health. For example, several studies have shown significant negative correlations between the PIL and the Minnesota Multiphasic Personality Inventory—Depression scale ($r = -.30$ to $-.65$, $p < .01$; Crumbaugh and Maholick 1964; Crumbaugh 1968; Crumbaugh and Maholick 1981), and significant positive correlations have been reported between the PIL and the self-acceptance ($r = .40$, $p < .01$), sense of well-being ($r = .52$, $p < .01$), achievement via conformance ($r = .63$, $p < .01$), and psychological mindedness ($r = .47$, $p < .01$) subscales of the California Psychological Inventory (CPI; Bonebright et al. 2000). The PIL is also negatively correlated with the Srole Anomie Scale ($r = -.48$ for males and $r = -.32$ for females, $p < .05$; Srole 1956), suggesting that the concept of the existential vacuum and anomie, or a lack of social norms, may overlap (Crumbaugh 1968).

The PIL has been subjected to more tests of psychometric soundness than any other measure of purpose. In sum, the measure appears to be a reliable measure of the degree of personal meaning present among both adult (Crumbaugh 1968; Crumbaugh and Maholick 1967; Guttman 1996; Meier and Edwards 1974; Reker 1977) and adolescent samples (Sink et al. 1998). For example, Sink et al. (1998) administered the 20-item PIL to samples of rural and urban adolescents and reported Cronbach's alpha values of .88 and .86, respectively. One-week retest reliability coefficients have been found to range from .68 to .83 ($p < .01$, Meier and Edwards 1974; Reker 1977). A 6-week retest coefficient of .79 ($p < .001$, Reker and Cousins 1979) and 8-week retest coefficients of .66 among rural and .78 among urban samples have also been reported (no p-values reported; Sink et al. 1998). Reliability estimates among adult samples are similar to those reported with adolescents (Guttman 1996). Spearman-Brown Corrected split-halt reliability coefficients ranging from .76 to .85 corrected by the Spearman-Brown formula to .87 and .92 have been obtained in four different studies with adults (Crumbaugh 1968; Crumbaugh and Maholick 1964; Hutzell 1988; Reker 1977; Reker and Cousins 1979).

Among adult samples, the PIL also appears to be valid measure of Frankl's will to meaning concept (Chamberlain and Zika 1988; Crumbaugh 1968; Crumbaugh and Henrion 1988; Crumbaugh and Maholick 1967; Hutzell 1988; Reker 1977). Construct validity has been supported by various comparisons of group means of different populations (Crumbaugh and Maholick 1981). Consistent with Frankl's theory, low PIL scores are significantly associated with suicide ideation (Harlowe et al. 1986; Kinnier et al. 1994), psychopathology (Kish and Moody 1989), depression and anxiety (Schulenberg 2004), and drug use (Harlowe et al. 1986; Kinnier et al. 1994; Padelford 1974), while high PIL scores predict positive self-concept, self-esteem, internal locus of control, life satisfaction, and planning (Reker 1977). In fact, because many of the PIL's questions probe happiness, some have argued that the PIL may actually be an indirect measure of life satisfaction (Damon et al. 2003) or an inverse measure of depression (Dyck 1987; Schulenberg 2004; Steger 2006; Yalom 1980). However, positive correlations between purpose and indicators of well-being and negative correlations between purpose and depression are never perfect, suggesting that the PIL is assessing a related but distinct construct.

Questions have also arisen with regards to the dimensionality of the life purpose construct measured by the PIL. Some researchers, using exploratory and confirmatory factor analysis, have concluded that the measure only assesses a single factor when certain items are excluded (Dale 2002; Marsh et al. 2003). Others have argued that it is clearly multidimensional. For instance, based on a qualitative review of the items, Yalom (1980) suggested that the survey assessed six different constructs, including purpose, life satisfaction, freedom, fear of death, suicidal thoughts, and how worthwhile one perceives one's life to be. Others have used factor analytic techniques to identify distinct dimensions. For instance, Shek (1988) concluded that the measure consists of five dimensions, including feelings regarding one's quality of life, goals, death, choices, and retirement. Still others have argued that it features only two dimensions, but they disagree on what those two dimensions are. Using exploratory factor analysis, one team of researchers concluded that the measure assessed an affective (sum of items 3, 4, 13, 17, 18, and 20) and a cognitive dimension, (sum of items 1, 2, 5, 6, 8, 9, 11, 12, 16, and 19) (Dufton and Perlman 1986; Shek 1993; Shek et al. 1987), while other researchers concluded it assesses an exciting life (items 2, 5, 7, 10, 17–19) and a purposeful life (items 3, 8, 20; Morgan and Farsides 2009). As a result of these contradictory findings, simply creating a composite score, if they do not assess a single factor, is likely to compromise the reliability and validity of the results and consequently has been cautioned against (Marsh et al. 2003). Additional assessments of the measure with a wider range of participants are clearly needed.

In part as a means of addressing the dimensionality issues raised with the full-length PIL, a shortened version was recently proposed. The Purpose in Life—Short Form (PIL-SF; Schulenberg et al. 2011) includes four of the PIL items that, according to confirmatory factor analytic techniques, fit well together. These four items focus primarily on goal attainment (questions 3, 4, 8, and 20). The internal consistency reliability coefficient alpha for the 20-item PIL was .86 and for the independently administered 4-item PIL-SF it was .84, suggesting that the short version is as reliable as the long one (Schulenberg et al. 2011). When administered separately, responses to the short form correlated with responses on the full PIL (r=.75, p<.01, 1-tailed), and similar to the PIL, scores on the PIL-SF also correlate positively with scores on measures of psychological well-being and negatively with scores on measures of psychological distress. The PIL-SF appears to represent a viable alternative to the full PIL, but it has rarely been used in empirical research.

The PIL, on the other hand, continues to be used regularly with adolescent (Sink et al. 1998) and adult samples (Crumbaugh 1968; Crumbaugh and Maholick 1967; Guttman 1996; Meier and Edwards 1974; Reker 1977), but it has not frequently been administered to younger individuals. This is likely because some items are inappropriate for early adolescents. For instance, items regarding the clarity of life goals may be too abstract for early adolescents, questions probing the reasons for existence may be beyond the lived experience of early adolescents, and items about death likely represent issues that most early adolescents do not regularly consider. Therefore, researchers interested in assessing purpose among early adolescents selected only the PIL items that were relevant to the lives of youth and created an Existence Subscale of Purpose in Life Test (EPIL; Law 2012). The 7-items of the EPIL focus on enthusiasm and excitement about life, a belief that daily activities are worthwhile, and a conviction that life has meaning. The creators of the measure conducted an assessment of the scale's psychometric properties with 2,842 early adolescents (Law 2012). They obtained a Cronbach's alpha value of .89. Exploratory factor analysis identified one factor that accounted for 60 % of the variance, and the factor structure was stable across genders. To assess the measures criterion-related validity, it was successfully used to differentiate volunteers from non-volunteers, whereby early adolescent volunteers scored higher on the EPIL than early adolescent youth who were not involved in volunteer activity. Though these findings suggest that the EPIL could be a useful measure of purpose among early adolescents, it has rarely been used in empirical studies. Of course, that may be because the measure is still relatively new.

Similar to the EPIL, the Life Purpose Questionnaire (LPQ; Hablas and Hutzell 1982; Hutzell 1989) represents another variation on the PIL; however, this one has been more widely administered. Because the PIL uses different response anchors for each question, researchers have argued that it may be confusing for some participants (Harlow et al. 1986; Schulenberg 2004). Therefore, the LPQ was developed as an uncomplicated, easily administered, paper-and-pencil measure of life meaning and purpose. Like the PIL, this measure includes 20-items that assess aspects of purpose and meaning, but unlike the PIL it includes statements, rather than phrases, to which participants respond using a simple dichotomous-choice format (*agree—disagree*). The LPQ was designed for use with specialized populations of individuals who are likely to be confused by the PIL, including geriatric participants, neuropsychiatric inpatients, alcoholics, and individuals with other special needs (Hablas and Hutzell 1982; Hutzell and Peterson 1986).

Among adults, the LPQ appears to be a psychometrically sound measure of purpose (Hablas and Hutzell 1982). Correlations between the LPQ and the PIL have been found to range from .60 to .80 (Hutzell 1989; Kish and Moody 1989), and, similar to the PIL, scores on the LPQ correlate positively with life satisfaction and negatively with depression (Hutzell 1989). However, psychometric properties of the LPQ have not been as thoroughly investigated as psychometric properties of the PIL, and additional assessments have been called for (Kish and Moody 1989). In spite of this, the measure does appear to be a useful for assessing purpose among special populations that struggle to understand the more confusing PIL response options (Hutzell 1989). In fact, respondents report that they prefer taking the LPQ to the PIL (Schulenberg 2004).

The Life Purpose Questionnaire has also been adapted for use with adolescents (Hutzell and Finck 1994). The measure omits two items that are not relevant to younger participants (Item seven: "Retirement means a time for me to do some of the exciting things I have always wanted to do." Item 15: "I am not prepared for death.") The remaining 18 items in the Life Purpose Questionnaire—Adolescent version (LPQ-A; Hutzell and Finck 1994) include questions such as the following, "I am often bored," "I have definite ideas of the things I want to do," and "My life is meaningful." Respondents agree or disagree with each of the statements. The measure has been used to assess life purpose among young people undergoing alcohol and drug treatment.

The LPQ-A measure has not been used much in empirical research. As such, its psychometric properties have rarely been investigated beyond the limited assessments conducted by its authors (Hutzell and Finck 1994). As a means of assessing the measure, Hutzell and Finck administered it to two groups of adolescents: one group consisted of youth in a support group for drug and alcohol use ($n = 100$) and the other group included more typical youth ($n = 100$). Each of the 18-items in the measure was correlated with the total score of the remaining items, and correlations ranged from .21 to .55 for the support group, averaging .37, and from .23 to .62 for the more typical group, averaging .48. Since this measure is based on Frankl's theory regarding the centrality of purpose to human well-being, the authors expected to find that the typical group would score higher than the support group. Results confirmed this hypothesis. The support group mean score was 10.6 (SD = 4.1) while the typical group mean score was 12.5 (SD = 4.5), and this difference was statistically significant ($t(198) = 3.13$; p two-tailed $< .01$).

The Purpose In Life Scale (PILS; Robbins and Francis 2000) represents yet another measure of purpose based largely on the PIL. This unidimensional measure consists of 12-items, including the following, "My life seems most worthwhile," "I feel my life has a sense of purpose," and "My life has clear goals and aims." Participants respond via a 5-point Likert scale ("1: strongly disagree" to "5: strongly agree.") Psychometric properties of the PILS were assessed among a sample of 517 undergraduate students. A Cronbach's alpha value of .90 was obtained, and high scores on the measure were found to to be associated with church attendance

($r=.11$, $p<.001$), stable extraversion ($r=.23$, $p<.001$), and low levels of neuroticism ($r=-.35$, $p<.001$) (Robbins and Francis 2000).

In addition to helping develop the PIL, Crumbaugh later developed the Seeking of Noetic Goals Test (SONG) as a complement to the PIL. Just as the PIL assesses the degree to which individuals have *found* a purpose for their lives, the SONG assesses the degree to which individuals are actively *searching* for a purpose for their lives (Crumbaugh 1977).

The SONG represents the earliest measure of record to assess the search for purpose. The motivation to find purpose is referred to by Frankl as *noetic,* or the spiritual, inspirational, aspirational, or non-material aspects of life. Frankl believed people should be motivated to search for a larger meaning for their lives. However, in spite of Frankl's focus on issues beyond-the-self, items in the SONG do not directly assess these kinds of concerns. Instead, items include the following: "I think about the ultimate meaning in life," "I am restless," and "I feel that some element which I cannot quite define is missing from my life." Responses are scaled on a seven point Likert scale (from "1: never" to "7: constantly").

Several researchers have assessed the psychometric properties of the SONG (e.g. Crumbaugh 1977; Melton and Schulenberg 2008; Reker and Cousins 1979). Reported Cronbach alpha coefficients range from .81 to .84, and 6 and 8-week retest reliabilities range from .66 to .78 (no *p*-values reported in either study; Reker and Cousins 1979; Sink et al. 1998). The SONG appears to distinguish between patient and non-patient groups whereby, as would be expected based on Frankl's will to meaning assumption, psychiatric patients are less motivated to search for purpose than non-patient adults (Crumbaugh 1977).

According to Crumbaugh (1977), scores on the PIL and SONG questionnaires should be inversely related since people with a purpose in their lives should not be motivated to search for one. As Crumbaugh (1977) predicted, SONG scores are significantly negatively correlated with PIL scores ($r=-.33$, $p<.001$; Reker and Cousins 1979). Further, using ten dimensions of life satisfaction, researchers (Reker and Cousins 1979) determined that items loaded on six factors in the PIL and on four factors in the SONG, suggesting again that the PIL and SONG function, as intended, as complementary measures. However, Crumbaugh (1977) proposed that the search for purpose and the presence of purpose were *always* inversely related, and this does not appear to be the case. Assessments using different measures of purpose have concluded that the search for purpose and the presence of purpose appear to be inversely related among adults, but not among adolescents (Bronk et al. 2009; Steger and Kashdan 2007). To date the PIL and SONG have not been administered together to adolescent samples. The relationship between the identification of purpose and the search for purpose is elaborated upon more fully in Chap. 7 (The Experience of Purpose among Diverse Groups).

The Life Attitude Profile-Revised (LAP-R; Reker 1992) is yet another survey measure based on Frankl's (1978) Will to Meaning assumption. It is a multidimensional measure designed to assess both current levels of purpose and the motivation to find purpose. The original LAP (Reker and Peacock 1981; Reker et al. 1987) included 56 items, but revisions resulted in a 48-item measure that is conceptually tighter and composed of an equal number of items per dimension (Reker 1992). The LAP-R consists of six dimensions including, purpose, coherence, choice/responsibility, death acceptance, existential vacuum, and goal seeking. Two composite scales are derived from these dimensions: the personal meaning index (purpose + coherence) and existential transcendence (purpose + coherence + choice/responsibility + death acceptance minus existential vacuum + goal setting). The six LAP-R dimensions have been shown to be internally consistent, stable over time, and valid measures of their respective constructs (Reker 1992). Questions in the LAP-R include, "My past achievements have given my life meaning and purpose" and "I feel that some element which I can't quite define is missing from my life." Participants respond to these questions via a 7-point Likert scale ("1: strongly disagree" to "7: strongly agree"), and scores correlate significantly with PIL scores, Life Regard Index-Revised Framework scores, and ratings of meaningfulness (Reker 1992).

Measures such as the LAP-R were designed for use with more typical respondents, but similar measures have also been created for use with more specialized groups of individuals. Frankl believed that challenges and even suffering presented opportunities to discover a purpose in life, and based on this premise, Patricia Starck (1983) created the Meaning in Suffering Test (MIST; Starck 1983, 1985) which assesses levels of meaning in life specifically related to unavoidable suffering. The MIST has two parts. The second part is primarily used for gathering potentially useful information for therapy (Starck 1985), but it is difficult to quantify (Schulenberg 2004) and as such is not frequently used in research. The first part, however, is composed of 20-items including, "I believe suffering causes a person to find new and more worthwhile life goals," and "I believe everyone has a purpose in life; a reason for being on Earth." Responses are scored on a 7-point Likert scale ("1: never" to "7: constantly"). The measure consists of three subscales: subjective characteristics of suffering, personal response to suffering items, and meaning in suffering (Starck 1985). MIST scores among nursing students and hospitalized patients correlate significantly with scores of other measures of purpose and related constructs (Guttman 1996; Schulenberg 2004; Starck 1985).

The MIST has not been used extensively in empirical studies, but a fairly recent investigation reveals that while total MIST scores demonstrate acceptable internal consistency (Cronbach's alpha = .83), two of the measure's three subscales demonstrate low internal consistency (Cronbach's alpha = .52 for the 6-item subjective experience of suffering subscale and Cronbach's apha = .53 for the 8-item personal responses to suffering subscale; Schulenberg 2004). As such, when using the MIST in research it is advisable to use the total score rather than the subscale scores (Schulenberg et al. 2006).

Finally, the last measure of purpose based on Frankl's conception of the construct is the Revised Youth Purpose Survey (Bundick et al. 2006). While measures exist that assess both identified purpose and the search for purpose, and measures exist to assess purpose among both adult and adolescent populations, this is the first measure that assesses both identified purpose and the search for purpose among adolescents. In addition to drawing from the PIL, items in this measure are also adapted from other existing measures of purpose (Ryff's Scales of Psychological

Well-being; Ryff and Keyes 1995) and meaning (Meaning in Life Questionnaire; Steger et al. 2006). The multidimensional scale was designed to probe the search for purpose, the presence of purpose, active engagement in working toward purpose, and the centrality or significance of purpose. However, repeated use of the survey reveals that these four components can be collapsed into two subscales: an Identified Purpose subscale (15 items; Cronbach's alpha=.94) and a Searching for Purpose subscale (5 items; Cronbach's alpha=.94; Bronk et al. 2009; Burrow et al. 2010). Participants rate the survey items on a seven-point Likert scale with higher scores indicating greater Identification and more Searching. "I have discovered a satisfying life purpose," is an Identified subscale item and "I am seeking a purpose or mission for my life" is a Searching subscale item.

As previously discussed, scores on the Searching and Identified subscales are positively correlated among adolescents and emerging adults, but not among midlife adults. In other words, adolescents who report having a purpose in life also tend to report searching for one, but consistent with the PIL and SONG relationship, midlife adults who have a purpose in life do not report searching for one (Bronk et al. 2009). Unfortunately, the PIL and SONG have not been administered to adolescent and young adult samples, but the emerging pattern of results suggests that the relationship between searching for and having identified a life purpose may be developmental in nature. This possibility is elaborated upon in greater detail in Chap. 4 (Purpose across the Lifespan). The Revised Youth Purpose survey is a relatively new measure, and as a result, it should be subjected to additional tests of psychometric soundness.

Ryff's Purpose in Life Sub-Scale

Behind Crumbaugh and Maholick's PIL test, Ryff's Purpose in Life subscale is the second most widely administered measure of purpose (Pinquart 2002). Ryff was an early advocate for empirical research on positive human health. She conceptualizes psychological well-being as consisting of six dimensions: autonomy, environmental mastery, personal growth, positive relations with others, self-acceptance, and life purpose (Ryff and Singer 1998). Called the Scales of Psychological Well-being, her self-report inventory is designed to assess an individual's welfare at a particular moment in time in each of these six areas. Subscales can be administered all together or on their own. The purpose in life subscale includes 20-, 14-, 9-, and 3-item versions. Individuals are asked to respond to questions such as, "I live life one day at a time and don't really think about the future (reverse scored)," and "Some people wander aimlessly through life, but I am not one of them." Responses are scaled from 1–6 on a Likert scale, with higher scores indicating the presence of more goals, greater direction in life, and a stronger purpose. Repeated assessments of the 20-item version reveal Cronbach alpha values ranging from .88 to .90 and a 6-week retest reliability score of .82 (Ryff 1989; Ryff et al. 1994, 2003). The 3-item scale was developed for use with telephone surveys, but it is not been found to be internally consistent (Ryff and Keyes 1995).

Antonovsky's Sense of Coherence Survey

Antonovsky's widely administered Sense of Coherence Scale (SOC; 1983) measures a construct similar to purpose. Commonly used in medical research, the SOC was developed to assess "salutogenesis," or the origins of health. More specifically, the SOC gauges the degree to which individuals believe their lives are comprehensible, manageable, and meaningful. Taken together, these beliefs support useful coping mechanisms, and individuals who hold these beliefs are likely to effectively manage stressful situations and stay well. Questions in the SOC include, "How often do you have the feeling that there is little meaning in the things you do in your daily life?"; "Do you have very mixed-up feelings and ideas?"; and "Do you have the feeling that you are in an unfamiliar situation and don't know what to do?" There are at least 15 versions of the SOC (Eriksson and Lindstrom 2005), but the most common versions are the original 29-item version (in which participants respond on a 7-point Likert scale) and a 13-item version (which uses the same response scale and includes a subset of the questions from the longer survey; Jakobsson 2011). While it might be tempting to use the meaning component of the SOC on its own, Antonovsky (1987) warned against this, saying it was intended for use as a measure of dispositional coping comprising all three subscales and its psychometric properties only apply to the full scale.

In 2005, researchers (Eriksson and Lindstrom) conducted a rigorous review of nearly 500 scientific publications featuring the SOC. They determined that in 124 studies using the measure, Cronbach's alpha values ranged from 0.70 to 0.95 and that retest correlations ranged from 0.69 to 0.78 over 1 year, from 0.59 to 0.67 over 5 years, and 0.54 over 10 years. They also concluded that SOC scores typically increase with age. Psychometric problems have arisen with shortened versions of the SOC (e.g. in a study of 1,753 participants, the 13-item version failed to show acceptable construct validity; Jakobsson 2011).

Like Antonovsky's "salutogenic" approach (1987), the Life Regard Index (LRI; Battista and Almond 1973) similarly assesses the degree to which life is viewed as meaningful and comprehensible. In particular, it measures the extent to which individuals demonstrate a positive regard for life, which Battista and Almond (1973) define as "an individual's belief that he is fulfilling his life as it is understood in terms of his highly valued life-framework of life-goals" (p. 413). The LRI is a self-report questionnaire composed of two subscales. The Framework subscale (LRI-FR) assesses the degree to which individuals can envision their lives within a meaningful perspective or have derived a set of life-goals, and the Fulfillment subscale (LFR-FU) measures the degree to which individuals see themselves as having fulfilled or as being in the process of fulfilling their framework or life goals.

The LRI includes 28 items. Half of the statements are phrased positively ("I have a clear idea of what I'd like to do with my life") and half are phrased negatively ("I don't really value what I'm doing"). In its original form the survey asked participants to respond on a five-point Likert scale, but Debats (LRI-R; 1998) suggested a new three-point Likert scale to avoid extreme responses ("1: I disagree," "2: I have no opinion," or "3: I agree").

The LRI has been subjected to a number of tests of psychometric soundness (e.g. Battista and Almond 1973; Chamberlain and Zika 1988; Debats et al. 1993, 1995). Cronbach's alpha values for the full LRI range from .87 to .91 depending on the sample (e.g. Cronbach's alpha = .87 among typical students; Cronbach's alpha = .91 among distressed students; Cronbach's alpha = .91 among general population sample). Reported internal consistency scores were similar for the two subscales (Cronbach's alpha LRI-FR = .84 among general population sample and Cronbach's alpha LRI-FU = .87; Debats et al. 1993). Five-week retest reliabilities for were calculated using Spearman's *rho* and yielded a coefficient of 0.80 (LRI), 0.73 (LRI-FR), and 0.79 (LRI-FU). Scores do not differ significantly either for the measure as a whole or for the subscales based on educational level or sex. However, married individuals do report significantly higher LRI scores than never married ($t = 3.43$, (130), $p < .001$) and divorced individuals ($t = 3.56$, (156), $p < .001$). To establish the construct validity of the LRI, the measure was correlated with a measure of happiness ($r = .73$, $p < .001$), depression ($r = -59$, $p < .001$), anxiety ($r = -.40$, $p < .001$), and general psychological distress ($r = -.52$, $p < .001$). Lastly, similar to other PIL measures, the LRI differentiates between typical and distressed samples, whereby typical individuals report higher life regard scores than do distressed individuals ($t = 10.8$ (269), $p < .001$, $d = 1.36$; Debats et al. 1993).

In a mixed-methods assessment of the LRI, researchers had participants complete the survey and respond to open-ended questions regarding specific experiences of meaning and meaninglessness. Results suggest that individuals who score high on positive life regard (as measured by the LRI) are more likely to describe experiences of meaningfulness with a variety of people including family, friends, and strangers, in which positive interactions, such as helping, and caring correspond with enjoying life fully and experiencing a sense of well-being (Debats et al. 1995). The authors conclude that meaningfulness, as assessed by the LRI, manifests as a state of positive engagement with others. Given this, and given lack the of goal orientation and beyond-the-self commitment, this measure appears to assess a construct more akin to meaning than purpose.

However, a multidimensional measure of purpose based in part on the LRI was recently proposed. Called the Meaningful Life Measure (MLM; Morgan and Farsides 2009), this survey actually assesses a construct more similar to purpose than meaning since it is composed of select items from the LRI, PIL, and Ryff's Psychological Well-being purpose subscale. This 23-item measure includes goal-oriented probes such as the following: "I have a clear idea of what my future goals and aims are," and "I tend to wander aimlessly through life, without much sense of purpose or direction" (reverse scored). Participants respond via a 7-point Likert scale ("1: strongly disagree" to "7: strongly agree"). Exploratory factor analysis reveals that the measure yields five factors, including, the exciting life, the accomplished life, the principled life, the purposeful life, and the valued life. Two of these factors, the purposeful life and the valued life, most closely assess life purpose as it has been conceived of in this book. The principled life measures understanding, the accomplished life gauges responsibility, and the exciting life captures enjoyment.

Preliminary assessments, with a sample composed primarily of college females, suggest that the measure is psychometrically sound. Alpha coefficients for the five subscales range from .85 to .88, and 6-month retest coefficients range from .64 to .70 (Morgan and Farsides 2009). However, additional studies are needed to confirm that the measure is reliable with a wider range of participants. Additional tests are also needed to assess the measure's convergent and discriminant validity.

Survey Measures of Meaning and Constructs Related to Purpose

Another cluster of measures assesses constructs closely related to purpose. For example, the Sources of Meaning Profile (SOMP; Reker and Wong 1988) measures the source and degree of personal meaning in one's life at different ages. The SOMP includes 16-items, and participants are asked to indicate on a seven-point Likert scale how important each potential source of meaning is to them. Potential sources of meaning include participating in leisure activities, leaving a legacy for the following generation, and serving others. The 16-item measure has yielded Cronbach alpha values of .77 and .78 (Reker 1988; Prager 1996) and a 3-month retest reliability coefficient of .70 (Reker 1988; Prager 1996).

In contrast to the SOMP, which assesses psychologists' theoretical ideas regarding what *should* represent individuals' sources of life meaning, the Personal Meaning Profile (PMP; Wong 1998) assesses laypeople's implicit theories of what actually *does* make their lives meaningful. Originally, this self-report measure consisted of 59-items, but following a revision it was cut down to 57-items that assess seven sources of life meaning, including achievement/striving (16 items), relationships (9 items), religion (9 items), transcendence (8 items), self-acceptance (6 items), intimacy (5 items) and fair treatment (4 items). These factors represent individuals' implicit theories of what makes life meaningful in practice as well as under ideal circumstances. The measure assesses the magnitude or intensity of life meaning (the greater the overall score, the more successful a person is in approximating the ideally meaningful life), the breadth of meaning (individuals who seek meaning from a variety of sources have a broader basis than individuals who derive meaning from only one or two sources), and balance (participants who score roughly equivalent across dimensions of meaning demonstrate a more balanced approach to life meaning). Research finds that self-ratings correlate with prototypical ratings and with criterion scores, suggesting that individuals who score higher on the PMP are closer to approximating an ideally meaningful life. Questions in the PMP include the following, "I have found someone I love deeply," and "I attempt to leave behind a good and lasting legacy." Participants respond to these questions via a seven-point Likert scale ("1: not at all" to "7: a great deal"). While the PMP's conception of meaning shares with purpose a focus on personal significance, it differs in that it lacks both future directedness and a commitment to the broader world.

The Meaning in Life Questionnaire represents another regularly administered measure of meaning (MLQ; Steger et al. 2006). This ten-item survey tool includes two five-item subscales: a searching for meaning subscale and a presence of meaning subscale. All items are scored on a seven-point Likert scale from "1: absolutely untrue" to "7: absolutely true." A sample Searching item includes, "I am always searching for something that makes my life feel significant," and a sample Presence item includes, "I understand my life's meaning." Recent use of this measure yielded a Cronbach alpha value of .80 (Yeagar and Bundick 2009). The measure is valid to the extent that it positively relates to a variety of measures of well-being, including life satisfaction and positive affect, and negatively relates to depression (Steger et al. 2006; Steger and Kashdan 2007).

Whereas the Meaning in Life Questionnaire assesses relatively stable feelings of meaning, a nearly identical measure, the Daily Meaning Scale (DMS; Steger et al. 2008; Stillman et al. 2009) assesses how participants feel "right now." Like the Meaning in Life Questionnaire, the Daily Meaning Scale includes both a Presence subscale (e.g. "Right now, how meaningful does your life feel?" 5-item, Cronbach's alpha=.78) and a Searching subscale (e.g. "How much are you searching for meaning in your life?" 5-item, Cronbach's alpha=.92), both of which are scored on a 7-point Likert scale, "1: not at all" to "7: absolutely."

Less Commonly Used Survey Measures of Purpose

Another cluster of research tools conflates purpose with other constructs. For example, the Values in Action Inventory of Strengths (VIA) is a self-report survey that assesses a range of potential personal strengths. Designed to help individuals identify their particular combination of character strengths, this survey includes two versions, one for adults 18 years of age and older (VIA—IS; Peterson and Seligman 2004) and one for youth between 10 and 17 years of age (VIA—Youth; Dahlsgaard 2005). Using exploratory factor analysis, the 24 strengths can be collapsed into four groups, including strengths of temperance, wisdom, interpersonal functioning, and transcendence. Transcendent strengths include purpose. However, because purpose is lumped in with other transcendent strengths, including spirituality and gratitude, its scores are not typically reported alone.

The Inventory of Positive Psychological Attitudes (IPPA; Kass et al. 1991) represents another positive psychology scale that includes a purpose in life dimension. This 30-item questionnaire taps two domains, purpose/life satisfaction and self-confidence in potentially stressful situations. The inventory scales were developed using factor analysis and Kass et al. (1991) report Cronbach's alpha values ranging from .88 to .94 for the total IPPA scale. Positive correlations between the IPPA scale and affect balance ($r=.66$, $p<.0001$) and between the IPPA scale and self-esteem ($r=.79$, $p<.0001$) and negative correlations between the IPPA scale and loneliness ($r = -.63$, $p < .0001$) have also been obtained. An empirical study using the measure suggests that positive changes in scores on this test correlate with positive changes in the health status of individuals who suffer from chronic pain (Kass et al. 1991). Both of these measures, the VIA and the IPPA, combine purpose with other constructs, and therefore are not useful measures of purpose alone. However, their existence underscores the central role of purpose in assessing physical and psychological well-being.

Other measures of purpose have been administered in professional, rather than research, contexts. For example, the Developing Purposes Inventory (Barratt 1978) is based on Chickering and Reisser's Seven Vectors of Student Development. Created in 1969 (Chickering 1969) and updated in 1993 (Chickering and Reisser 1993), this model of college student growth was designed to assess emerging adults' growth in seven key areas, including: developing competence, managing emotions, moving through autonomy toward interdependence, developing mature interpersonal relationships, establishing identity, developing integrity, and developing purpose (Chickering and Reisser 1993). The "developing purpose" vector assesses students' reasons for attending college and for choosing particular careers. It also measures students' personal aspirations, their commitments to family and other aspects of their lives, and their ability to balance these commitments (Chickering and Reisser 1993).

Barratt (1978) created the Developing Purposes Inventory (DPI) to assess the degree to which students were committed to pursuing a life purpose. His measure consists of three 15-item sub-scales (45 items total) designed to measure each of Chickering and Reisser's (1993) three sub-vectors of developing purpose, including avocational or recreational purpose, vocational or professional purpose, and lifestyle or interpersonal purpose. Sample questions include the following: "I attend special lectures and programs that are about my recreational interests" (avocational purpose); "I read the items that have been suggested or recommended by an instructor for a class but are not required" (professional or career purpose); and "I think about how my personal values relate to my career plans" (lifestyle purpose). Students use a five-point Likert scale ("1: never true" to "5: always true") to indicate how true each statement is for them.

Another tool designed to assess aspects of Chickering's theory of psychosocial development is the Student Developmental Task and Lifestyle Assessment (SDTLA; Winston 1990; Winston et al. 1999). Similar to the Developing Purposes Inventory, this measure has rarely been used in research, but has more often been used by student affairs professionals to help students understand and reflect upon their growth, to assist them in setting goals and planning for the future, and to guide interventions (Winston 1990). As such, this measure is designed for use with college students between roughly 17 and 24 years of age. It is composed of 140 true–false questions, drawn from six general categories including the following: developing mature interpersonal relations, academic autonomy, salubrious lifestyle, intimacy, establishing and clarifying purpose, and response bias.

The *establishing and clarifying purpose* dimension is of greatest interest here. Of the 140 total questions, 68 assess this developmental task. Establishing and clarifying purpose consists of five subtasks. The first is Educational Involvement (EI; 16 items), which measures the extent to which students have thoroughly explored and identified well-defined goals for their educational experience and the extent to which they show signs of being self-directed, active learners. The second dimension, Career Planning (CP; 19 items), measures the degree to which students have devised a professional plan that takes into consideration their strengths and weaknesses and their educational background. It also reflects the degree to which students have emotionally committed to a career plan. The third dimension, Lifestyle Planning (LP; 11 items), assesses the extent to which students have identified a personal direction for their lives that takes into account their religious and moral beliefs along with their family and vocational plans. Fourth, this instrument assesses students' Life Management (LM; 16 items) skills, or the degree to which students organize their lives to satisfy their daily needs and to meet their personal and financial responsibilities. Finally, this tool measures students Cultural Participation (CIP; 6 items), or their range of cultural interests and level of participation in cultural activities.

Assessments of the *establishing and clarifying purpose* measure have been conducted in conjunction with the development of the measurement. Cronbach's alpha values for this 68-item subscale range from .45 to .90. Two-week retest scores range from .80 to .87, 4-week retest scores from .76 to .85, and 20-week retest scores from .53 to .73 (Winston and Miller 1987; Winston 1988). Investigations into validity reveal that items in the same sub-scale correlate more strongly with each other than with items in any of the other sub-scales; however, items in the academic autonomy sub-scale correlate relatively highly with items in the purpose sub-scale. The purpose sub-scale was also found to correlate positively with measures of study skills, career planning, and career exploration (Winston 1988).

Finally, the last less commonly used measure of purpose is a one-item survey. This measure asks participants, typically adolescents, to complete the following question, "I feel my life has a sense of purpose," using a 5-point Likert scale ("1: strongly agree" to "5: strongly disagree"; Francis 2000; Francis and Burton 1994; Francis and Evans 1996; Robbins and Francis 2000). This measure has not been administered frequently, given the limitations inherent in a single-item tool.

Taken together, studies utilizing the preceding survey measures of purpose have yielded considerable insight into our growing understanding of the construct both from research and practice perspectives. However, there is one significant problem with existing survey measures. None assesses the "other-oriented" dimension of the construct. None is able to discern whether individuals are motivated to pursue a purpose in life for reasons other than solely self-oriented ones, and this means that none of the existing survey measures is able to assess the full purpose construct. Designing a survey to achieve this task has proven challenging. To assess the illusive but essential beyond-the-self component of purpose, a survey would need to first establish what an individual found purposeful in his or her life and then probe why this aim was particularly meaningful. This multi-step task is more easily accomplished using other research tools. In particular, interviews, diary studies, and document reviews have proven to be useful ways of assessing the beyond-the-self dimension of the purpose construct.

Interview Protocols

Interviews are typically used to provide qualitative, "thick descriptions" of an experience (Geertz 1983). They can be used to flesh out quantitative findings and to develop hypotheses that can later be tested in survey research. In the case of purpose, they are particularly useful in shedding light on the motivations behind one's purposeful aims. Unlike surveys, they can be used to better understand individuals' reasons for pursuing personally meaningful aspirations.

In spite of the usefulness of interviews in assessing all the key dimensions of purpose, they are infrequently used. In fact, after a thorough review of the purpose literature, I was only able to identify one interview protocol designed to assess purpose and one designed to assess generativity, a concept related to purpose. The scarcity of interview protocols is likely the result of the time intensive and expensive nature of carrying out interview research.

The Revised Youth Purpose Interview (Andrews et al. 2006) is a semi-structured interview protocol derived from studies of self-understanding and identity development (see, for example, Colby and Damon 1993; Damon and Hart 1988; Hart and Fegley 1995). The protocol consists of two parts. The first part features a line of questioning designed to determine what is particularly important to the individual. Questions in this section include more general, open-ended probes, such as, "What are some of the things you really care about?" and "What matters to you most?" To encourage participants to think about concerns beyond themselves, questions also ask about issues that matter to participants in the broader world. A question along this line includes the following: "Imagine you've been given a magic wand and you can change anything you want in the world, what would you want to be different?" Once interviewees have identified the aim or aims that matter most to them, the interviewer begins the second half of the interview, which focuses on gaining a deeper understanding of the role this potential driver plays in the interviewee's life. So, for example, if the interviewee has said one of the most important aspirations in his or her life is to have a family or help others through a particular career, then the remainder of the interview would focus on understanding just how central this particular aim is, why it is as central as it is, and what steps the interviewee has taken or plans to take in order to make progress toward this aim.

The interview takes about an hour to administer and has typically been used with adolescent and emerging adult samples (Bronk 2005, 2008, 2011, 2012; Bronk et al. 2010; Damon 2008; Moran 2009; Yeagar and Bundick 2009). Findings from studies administering this protocol have revealed much about the prevalence of purpose among different samples of young people (Bronk et al. 2010; Damon 2008; Moran 2009), the role of purpose in healthy identity development (Bronk 2011), and role of meaning in school work and professional plans (Yeagar and Bundick

2009). This protocol has also been used to build a theory of the way purposes develop and change over time (Bronk 2012) and to highlight characteristics of youth with purpose (Bronk 2008). Finally, because the interview protocol is, at present anyway, one of the few reliable ways of determining the motivations behind one's purposeful pursuits, it has also been used to examine the impact of pursuing personal aspirations for self-serving and beyond-the-self reasons. In one such study, characteristics and indicators of youth thriving with self-oriented and other-oriented long-term aims were compared (Bronk and Finch 2010). Results revealed that youth with beyond the-self long term aims reported higher levels of life satisfaction than youth with self-serving aims.

The other relevant interview protocol, the Life Story Interview (McAdams 2008), was designed to gather information about, among other things, generativity among older adults. Generativity represents Erikson's seventh stage of psychosocial development, and it describes adults' level of concern with leaving behind a positive legacy and with making contributions to the broader world that will outlive themselves. For example, parenting or volunteering can be generative acts. In this way, generativity shares with purpose an important focus on beyond-the-self motivations.

The Life Story Interview takes approximately two hours to administer and is broken into eight sections. The first section focuses on the different chapters in the interviewees' life. The second section asks participants to discuss a variety of key scenes, including high points and low points, in their life story. Third, participants are asked to focus on the future and to discuss their hopes, dreams, and plans. In this section, participants are encouraged to discuss a life project, or "something that you have been working on and plan to work on in the future chapters of your life story. The project might involve your family or your work life, or it might be a hobby, avocation, or pastime" (McAdams 2008). Based on this description, a life project could represent a life purpose. Next, participants are encouraged to reflect on the challenges they have encountered in their lives. The sixth and seventh sections ask participants to reflect on their personal ideology, including their religious, moral, and political beliefs, and their life themes, respectively. Finally, the last section asks participants to reflect on the experience of being interviewed. Themes relevant to purpose and generativity are likely to surface in the life project interview section, but also throughout the interview.

Following is a table that includes a summary of the most commonly used survey and interview measures of purpose and closely related constructs.

Other Measures of Life Purpose

In addition to survey and interview measures, researchers have also utilized other means of assessing the purpose construct. Early in the study of purpose, Inhelder and Piaget (1958) reviewed the private diaries of a sample of twentieth-century

Instrument name	Description	Sample question
Survey measures of the presence of purpose and related constructs		
Existence of Purpose in Life subscale (EPIL; Law 2012) for early adolescence	7 items selected from the PIL based on their relevance to the lives of early adolescents	"My life is—(1) *empty* (7) *running over with good things*"
Life Profile Questionnaire (LPQ; Hablas and Hutzell 1982)	20 items very similar to PIL; agree/disagree format to aid comprehension in geriatric, neuro-psychiatric patient, and other special populations	"I am usually able to think of a usefulness to my life,"—*agree, disagree*
Life Purpose Questionnaire—Adolescent Version (LPQ-A; Hutzell and Finck 1994)	18 items; agree/disagree format to aid comprehension among adolescent participants	"I have discovered many reasons why I was born,"—*agree, disagree*
Meaning in Suffering Test (MIST; Starck 1983)	20 items, 7-point Likert response format; yields a total score and three subscale scores	"I believe my suffering experience has given me a chance to complete my mission in life,"—(1) *never* (7) *constantly*
Purpose in Life Scale (PILS; Robbins and Francis 2000)	12 items with a 5-point Likert response option	"My personal experience is full of direction,"—(1) *disagree strongly* (5) *agree strongly*
Purpose in Life Test (PIL; Crumbaugh 1968; Crumbaugh and Maholick 1964)	20 items, 7-point Likert response format; different anchoring points for each item, with 4 being neutral	"Life to me seems"—(1) *completely routine*—(7) *always exciting*
Purpose in Life Test—Short Form (PIL-SF; Schulenberg et al. 2011)	4-items drawn from the PIL, 7-point Likert response format; different anchoring points for each item, with 4 being neutral	"In life I have"—(1) *no clear goals*—(7) *clear goals and aims*
Ryff's Scales of Psychological Well-being Purpose Subscale (Ryff 1989; Ryff and Keyes 1995)	20, 14, 9, and 3 item versions with a 6-point Likert response option; unidimensional measure of purpose represents one of six dimensions of psychological well-being	"Some people wander aimlessly through life, but I am not one of them"—(1) *strongly disagree*—(6) *strongly agree*
Sense of Coherence Scale (SOC; Antonovsky 1983, 1987)	29 and 13 item versions administered most commonly; 7-point Likert response format	"Until now your life has had"—(1) *no clear goals*—(7) *very clear goals and purpose*

Instrument name	Description	Sample question
Survey measures of the motivation to find purpose		
Seeking of Noetic Goals (SONG; Crumbaugh 1977)	20 statements rated on a 7-point Likert response format; unidimensional scale of the motivation to find purpose	"I feel that some element which I cannot quite define is missing from my life"—(1) *never*—(7) *constantly*
Survey measures of purpose and the motivation to find purpose		
Daily Meaning Scale (DMS; Steger et al. 2008)	10 items, 7-point Likert response format; 2 subscales, Presence of meaning (5 items) and Searching for meaning (5 items)	"Right now, how meaningful does your life feel?"—(1) *not at all*—(7) *absolutely*
Life Attitude Profile—Revised (LAP-R; Reker and Peacock 1981; Reker 1992)	48 items, 7-point Likert response format; yields six dimension and two composite scores	"My past achievements have given my life meaning and purpose"—(1) *strongly disagree*—(7) *strongly agree*
Life Regard Index (LRI; Battista and Almond 1973; Debats et al. 1995)	28 items with two subscales; Framework subscale measures existence of life goals and Fulfillment subscale measures progress toward life goals	"I have a clear idea of what I'd like to do with my life"—*I disagree, I have no opinion, I agree*
Meaningful Life Measure (MLM; Morgan and Farsides 2009)	23 item measure composed of items from the LRI, PIL, and Ryff's Psychological Well-being Purpose subscale	"I have a clear idea of what my future goals and aims are"—(1) *strongly disagree*—(7) *strongly agree*
Meaning in Life Questionnaire (MLQ; Steger et al. 2006)	10 items, 7—point Likert response format; 2 subscales, Presence of meaning (5 items) and Searching for meaning (5 items)	"I understand my life's meaning"—(1) *absolutely untrue*—(7) *absolutely true*
Revised Youth Purpose Survey (Bundick et al. 2006)	20 items, 7-point Likert response format; 2 subscales, Identified purpose (15 items) and Searching purpose (5 items)	"My life has a clear sense of purpose" (identified), "I am always looking to find my life's purpose" (searching)—(1) *strongly disagree* to (7) *strongly agree*

Instrument name	Description	Sample question
Personal Meaning Profile (PMP; Wong 1998)	57 items, 7-point Likert response format; 7 dimensions including achievement, relationships, religion, self-transcendence, self-acceptance, intimacy, and fair treatment	"I am enthusiastic about what I do." "I make a significant contribution to society." (1) *not at all*—(7) *a great deal*
Sense of Meaning Profile (SOMP; Reker 1988; Prager 1996)	16 items, 7-point Likert response format; assesses source and degree of meaning	"Leaving a legacy for the next generation"—(1) *not at all important*—(7) *very important*
Interview measures		
Life Story Interview (McAdams 2008)	Semi-structured interview protocol that guides the participant through a telling of his or her life story, complete with chapters, characters, and themes. Includes a section on life projects	"A life project is something that you have been working on and plan to work on in the future chapters of your life story. The project might involve your family or your work life, or it might be a hobby, avocation, or pastime. Please describe any project that you are currently working on or plan to work on in the future. Tell me what the project is, how you got involved in the project or will get involved in the project, how the project might develop, and why you think this project is important for you and/or for other people."
Revised Youth Purpose Interview Protocol (Andrews et al. 2006)	Semi-structured interview protocol that probes the goals that matter most, the depth of commitment to these aims, the reasons behind these aims, and activity/plans for working toward them	"What are some of the things that really matter to you? Imagine you're 40 years of age, what will you be doing? What will be important to you? Why?"

adolescents in Switzerland. The essays, which were not written for public consumption, represent intimate documents. The researchers collected and reviewed them for other purposes, but they noted that the adolescents, without any prompting or encouragement, consistently discussed their hopes, dreams, and aspirations, and in so doing, frequently described various purposes. Despite the interesting and important findings regarding purpose and adolescent development more generally that resulted from this creative study, this approach has some limitations, including the great challenge presented in getting adolescents to share their personal and private musings with researchers. Beyond this, of course, this methodology precludes follow up questions, and does not allow for direct questioning of purpose. Bearing in mind these limitations, diary reviews clearly represent an interesting and potentially under-utilized approach to studying the purpose construct.

Another way purpose has been explored is through reviews of historical documents. Mariano and Valliant (2012) investigated adolescent and emerging adult purposes among the "greatest generation," or individuals who came of age during World War II. They reviewed health documents and interviews conducted with young men who served in World War II with the goal of identifying spontaneous references to purpose and beyond-the-self aspirations. While this approach yielded interesting findings regarding the nature of purpose among this generation, it suffers some of the same limitations as the diary review approach. These robust data sets are rare, expensive to compile, and preclude follow-up and direct questions about purpose.

Finally, DeVogler and Ebersole endeavored to identify the range of inspiring types of purpose or sources of meaning, and they employed a creative means of doing so. First, in the Meaning Essay Document, they asked participants to describe and rank their three most important sources of meaning and to list a concrete experience associated with each one (DeVogler and Ebersole 1980). The investigators had adolescents (1983), college students (1980), and adults (1981) complete this task, and what emerged was a useful classification of sources of meaning. The categories of meaning that emerged are discussed more fully in Chap. 6 ("Inspiring Types of Purpose").

Subsequent to developing the Meaning Essay Document, Ebersole and Sacco (1983) created the Meaning in Life Depth instrument (MILD). In contrast to their earlier line of inquiry, this measure aims not only to identify different sources of meaning in life, but also to assess the depth of commitment to each source of meaning, partially independent of respondent's self-reports. To complete the MILD, participants rank from most to least personally significant eight commonly identified sources of meaning, derived from DeVogler and Ebersole's earlier studies. Participants are also given the option of selecting "no meaning" for their lives. Next, respondents are asked to write a brief essay about how significant their most important source of meaning is. Judges are then recruited to read the essays and to assign a depth score, relative to the other essays. However, given that a third party ultimately assigns a meaning level, the approach has been criticized as biased (Ebersole and Kobayakawa 1989).

It is clear from this review, that a wide range of tools exists to assess the purpose construct. Of course, no single measure is perfect, but taken together surveys, interviews, and other more creative methodologies are yielding a rapidly emerging picture of purpose—what it is, how it functions, and why it is important. Among other things, empirical studies relying on these measures reveal that purpose plays a central role in optimal human functioning, and this topic is discussed in greater detail in the following chapter.

References

Andrews, M., Bundick, M., Jones, A., Bronk, K. C., Mariano, J. M., & Damon, W. (2006). *Revised youth purpose interview*. Unpublished instrument, Stanford Center on Adolescence, Stanford CA.

Antonovsky, A. (1983). *The sense of coherence scale*. Unpublished instrument, Ben-Gurion University, Israel.

Antonovsky, A. (1987). *Unraveling the mystery of health: How people manage stress and stay well*. San Francisco: Jossey-Bass.

Barrat, W. R. (1978). *Developing purposes inventory*. Iowa City: Hi Tech Press.

Battista, J., & Almond, R. (1973). The development of meaning in life. *Psychiatry, 36,* 409–427.

Bonebright, C. A., Clay, D. L., & Ankenmann, R. D. (2000). The relationship of workaholism with work-life conflict, life-satisfaction, and purpose in life. *Journal of Counseling Psychology, 47*(4), 469–477.

Bronk, K. C. (2005). Portraits of purpose: A grounded theory of the way purpose contributes to positive youth development. *Dissertation Abstracts International,* AAT 3187267.

Bronk, K. C. (2008). Humility among adolescent purpose exemplars. *Journal of Reseach on Character Education, 6*(1), 35–51.

Bronk, K. C. (2011). Portraits of purpose: The role of purpose in identity formation. A special issue on Instructing for and Supporting Youth Purpose in. *New Directions in Youth Development, 132,* 31–44.

Bronk, K. C. (2012). A grounded theory of youth purpose. *Journal of Adolescent Research, 27,* 78–109. http://dx.doi.org/10.1177/0743558411412958.

Bronk, K. C., & Finch, W. H. (2010). Adolescent characteristics by type of long-term aim in life. *Applied Developmental Science, 14*(1), 1–10.

Bronk, K. C., Hill, P., Lapsley, D., Talib, T., Finch, W. H. (2009). Purpose, hope, and life satisfaction in three age groups. *Journal of Positive Psychology, 4*(6), 500–510.

Bronk, K. C., Finch, W. H., & Talib, T. (2010). The prevalence of a purpose in life among high ability adolescents. *High Ability Studies, 21*(2), 133–145.

Bundick, M., Andrews, M., Jones, A., Mariano, J. M., Bronk, K. C., & Damon, W. (2006). *Revised youth purpose survey*. Unpublished instrument, Stanford Center on Adolescence, Stanford CA.

Burrow, A. L., O'Dell, A. C., & Hill, P. L. (2010). Profiles of a developmental asset: Youth purpose as a context for hope and well-being. *Journal of Youth and Adolescence, 39,* 1265–1273.

Chamberlain, K., & Zika, S. (1988). Religiosity, life meaning, and well-being: Some relationships in a sample of women. *Journal for the Scientific Study of Religion, 27,* 411–420.

Chickering, A. W. (1969). *Education and identity*. San Francisco: Jossey-Bass.

Chickering, A. W., & Reisser, L. (1993). *Education and identity* (2nd ed). San Francisco: Jossey-Bass.

Colby, A., & Damon, W. (1993). *Some do care: Contemporary lives of moral commitment*. New York: Free Press.

Crumbaugh, J. C. (1968). Cross-validation of Purpose in Life test based on Frankl's concepts. *Journal of Individual Psychology, 24,* 74–81.
Crumbaugh, J. C. (1977). The Seeking of Noetic Goals Test (SONG): A complimentary scale to the Purpose in Life Test (PIL). *Journal of Clinical Psychology, 33*(3), 900–907.
Crumbaugh, J. C., & Henrion, R. (1988). The PIL test: Administration, interpretation, uses, theory, and critiques. *The International Forum for Logotherapy, 11,* 76–88.
Crumbaugh, J. C., & Henrion, R. (2001). How to find meaning and purpose in life for the third millenium. *The International Forum for Logotherapy, 24,* 1–9.
Crumbaugh, J. C., & Maholick, L. T. (1964). An experimental study in existentialism: The psychometic approach to Frankl's concept of noogenic neurosis. *Journal of Clinical Psychology, 20,* 200–207.
Crumbaugh, J. C., & Maholick, L. T. (1967). An experimental study in existentialism: The psychometric approach to Frankl's concept of noogenic neurosis. In V. E. Frankl (Ed.), *Psychotherapy and existentialism* (pp. 183–197). New York: Washington Square Press.
Crumbaugh, J. C., & Maholick, L. T. (1981). *Manual of instructions for the Purpose in Life test.* Murfeesboro, TN: Psychometric Affiliates.
Dahlsgaard, K. (2005). Is virtue more than its own reward? *Dissertation Abstracts International: Section B: The Sciences and Engineering, 66*(6-B) (UMI No. AAI3179723).
Dale, A. (2002). *Do some drug users have less to live for*? Unpublished doctoral dissertation, School of Psychology, Curtin University of Technology, Western Australia.
Damon, W. (2008). *The path to purpose: Helping our children find their calling in life.* New York: The Free Press.
Damon, W., & Hart, D. (1988). *Self-understanding in childhood and adolescence.* Cambridge: Cambridge University Press.
Damon, W., Menon, J., & Bronk, K. C. (2003). The development of purpose during adolescence. *Applied Developmental Science, 7*(3), 119–128.
Debats, D. L. (1998). Measurement of personal meaning: The psychometric properties of the Life Regard Index. In P. T. P. Wong & P. S. Fry (Eds.), *The human quest for meaning: A handbook of psychological research and clinical application* (pp. 237–259). Mahwah: Erlbaum.
Debats, D. L., Van der Lubbe, P. M., & Wezeman, F. R. A. (1993). On the psychometric properties of the life regard index (LRI): A measure of meaningful life. *Personality and Individual Differences, 14,* 337–345.
Debats, D. L., Drost, J., & Hansen, P. (1995). Experiences if meaning in life: A combined qualitative and quantitative approach. *British Journal of Psychology, 86,* 359–375.
DeVogler, K. L., & Ebersole, P. (1980). Categorization of college students' meaning in life. *Psychological Reports, 46,* 387–390.
DeVogler, K. L., & Ebersole, P. (1981). Adults' meaning in life. *Psychological Reports, 49,* 87–90.
DeVogler, K. L., & Ebersole, P. (1983). Young adolescents'meaning in life. *Psychological Reports, 52,* 427–431.
Dufton, B. D., & Perlman, D. (1986). The association between religiosity and the Purpose in Life test (PIL): Does it reflect purpose or satisfaction? *Journal of Psychology and Theology, 14,* 42–48.
Dyck, M. J. (1987). Assessing logotherapeutic constructs: Conceptual and psychometric status of the purpose in life and seeking of noetic goals tests. *Clinical Psychology Review, 7*(4), 439–447.
Ebersole, P., & Kobayakawa, S. (1989). Bias in meaning in life ratings. *Psychological Reports, 65,* 911–914.
Ebersole, P., & Sacco, J. (1983). Meaning in life depth: Explicit ratings criteria. *Psychological Reports, 56,* 303–310.
Eriksson, M., & Lindstrom, B. (2005). Validity of Antonovsky's sense of coherence scale: A systematic review. *Journal of Epidemiology and Community Health, 59*(6), 460–466. doi:10.1136/jech.2003.018085.
Francis, L. J. (2000). The relationship between bible reading and purpose in life among 13- to 15-year olds. *Mental Health, Religion, and Culture, 3,* 27–36.

Francis, L. J., & Burton, L. (1994). The influence of personal prayer on purpose in life among Catholic adolescents. *The Journal of Beliefs and Values, 15*(2), 6–9.

Francis, L. J., & Evans, T. E. (1996). The relationships between personal prayer and purpose in life among churchgoing and non-churchgoing 12- to 15-year olds in the UK. *Religious Education, 91*(1), 9–21.

Frankl, V. E. (1959). *Man's search for meaning*. Boston: Beacon Press.

Geertz, C. (1983). Thick description: Toward an interpretive theory of culture. In R. M. Emerson (Ed.), *Contemporary field research*. Boston: Little, Brown.

Guttmann, D. (1996). *Logotherapy for the helping professional: Meaningful social work*. New York: Springer.

Hablas, R., & Hutzell, R. (1982). The Life Purpose Questionnaire: An alternative to the Purpose in Life test for geriatric, neuropsychiatric patients. In S. A. Wawrytko (Ed.), *Analecta Frankliana: The proceedings of the First World Congress of Logotherapy: 1980* (pp. 211–215). Berkeley: Strawberry Hill.

Harlowe, L., Newcomb, M., Bentler, P. (1986). Depression, self-derogation, substance abuse, and suicide ideation: Lack of purpose in life as a mediational factor. *Journal of Clinical Psychology, 42,* 5–21.

Hart, D., & Fegley, S. (1995). Prosocial behavior and caring in adolescence: Relations to self-understanding and social judgment. *Child Development, 66,* 1346–1359.

Hutzell, R. R. (1988). A review of the Purpose in Life test. *The International Forum for Logotherapy, 11,* 89–101.

Hutzell, R. R. (1989). *Life Purpose Questionnaire overview sheet*. Berkeley: Institute of Logotherapy Press.

Hutzell, R. R. (1995). Life purpose questionnaire. In L. L. Jeffries (Ed.), Adolescence and meaning in life (Doctoral dissertation, University of Houston, 1995). *Dissertation Abstracts International, 56,* O8B 4634.

Hutzell, R. R., & Finck, W. C. (1994). Adapting the life purpose questionnaire for use in adolescent populations. *The International Forum for Logotherapy, 17,* 42–46.

Hutzell, R. R., & Peterson, T. J. (1986). Use of the Life Purpose Questionnaire with an alcoholic population. *International Journal of the Addictions, 21*(1), 51–57.

Inhelder, B., & Piaget, J. (1958). *The growth of logical thinking from childhood to adolescence*. New York: Basic Books.

Jakobsson, U. (2011). Testing construct validity of the 13-item Sense of Coherence Scale in a sample of older people. *The Open Geriatric Medicine Journal, 4,* 6–13.

Jeffries, L. L. (1995). Adolescence and meaning in life. (Doctoral dissertation, University of Houston, 1995). *Dissertation Abstracts International, 56,* O8B 4634.

Jonsen, E., Fagerstrom, L., Lundman, B., Nygren, B., Vahakangas, M., & Strandberg, G. (2010). Psychometric properties of the Swedish version of the Purpose in life scale. *Scandinavian Journal of Caring Sciences, 24*(1), 41–8.

Kass, J. D., Friedman, R., Leserman, J., Caudill, M., Zuttermeister, P. C., & Benson, H. (1991). An Inventory of positive psycholgical attitudes with potential relevance to health outcomes: Validation and preliminary testing. *Behavioral Medicine, 17*(3), 121–129.

Kinnier, R., Metha, A. T., Keim, J. S., Okey, J. L., Adler-Tabia, R., Berry, M. A., & Mulvenon, S. W. (1994). Depression, meaninglessness, and substance abuse in "normal" and hospitalized adolescents. *Journal of Alcohol and Drug Education, 39*(2), 101–111.

Kish, G. B., & Moody, D. R. (1989). Psychopathology and life purpose. *The International Forum for Logotherapy, 12,* 40–45.

Kotchen, T. A. (1960). Existential mental health: An empirical approach. *Journal of Individual Psychiatry, 16,* 174–181.

Law, B. M. (2012). Psychometric properties of the existence subscale of the Purpose in Life questionnaire for Chinese adolescents in Hong Kong. *The Scientific World Journal,* Article ID 685741. doi:10.1100/2012/685741

Mariano, J. M., & Vaillant, G. E. (2012). Purpose among the "Greatest Generation." *Journal of Positive Psychology*. doi:10.1080/17439760.2012.686624.

Marsh, A., Smith, L., Piek, J., & Saunders, B. (2003). The Purpose in Life Scale: Psychometric properties for social drinkers and drinkers in alcohol treatment. *Educational and Psychological Measurement, 63*(5), 859–871.

McAdams, D. P. (2008). *The life story interview*. Retrieved May 22, 2012 from http://www.sesp.northwestern.edu/docs/LifeStoryInterview.pdf.

Melton, A. M. A., & Schulenberg, S. E. (2008). On the measurement of meaning: Logotherapy's empirical contributions to humanistic psychology. *The Humanistic Psychologist, 36,* 31–44.

Meier, A. & Edwards, H. (1974). Purpose in-life test: Age and sex differences. *Journal of Clinical Psychology,* 30, 384–386.

Moran, S. (2009). Purpose: Giftedness in intrapersonal intelligence. *High Ability Studies, 20*(2), 143–159.

Morgan, J., & Farsides, T. (2009). Measuring meaning in life. *Journal of Happiness Studies, 10,* 197–214.

Okado, T. (1998). *The Japanese version of the Purpose in Life test.* Tokyo: System Publica.

Padelford, B. (1974). Relationship between drug involvement and purpose in life. *Journal of Clinical Psychology, 30,* 303–305.

Peterson, C., & Seligman, M. E. P. (2004). *Character strengths and virtues: A handbook and classification.* New York: Oxford University Press.

Pinquart, M. (2002). Creating and maintaining purpose in life in old age: A meta-analysis. *Ageing International, 27*(2), 90–114.

Prager, E. (1996). Exploring personal meaning in an age-differentiated Australian sample: Another look at the Sources of Meaning Profile (SOMP). *Journal of Aging Studies, 10*(2), 117–136.

Reker, G. (1977). The Purpose in Life test in an inmate population: An empirical investigation. *Journal of Clinical Psychology, 33*(3), 688–93.

Reker, G. (1988). *Sources of personal meaning among middle-aged and other adults: A replication.* Paper presented at the Annual Meeting of the Gerontological Society of America. San Francisco.

Reker, G. (1992). *The Life Attitude Profile—Revised (LAP-R). Procedures manual: Research edition.* Peterborough: Student Psychologists Press.

Reker, G. T., & Cousins, J. B. (1979). Factor structure, construct validity and reliability of the Seeking of Noetic Goals (SONG) and Purpose in Life (PIL) tests. *Journal of Clinical Psychology, 35*(1), 85–91.

Reker, G. T., & Peacock, E. J. (1981). The life attitude profile (LAP): A multidimensional instrument for assessing attitudes toward life. *Canadian Journal of Behavioral Science, 13,* 64–73.

Reker, G. T., & Wong, P. T. P. (1988). Aging as an individual process: Toward a theory of personal meaning. In J. E. Birren & V. L. Bengston (Eds.), *Emergent theories of aging* (pp. 214–246). New York: Springer.

Reker, G. T., Peacock, E. J., & Wong, P. T. P. (1987). Meaning and purpose in life and well-being: A life-span perspective. *Journal of Gerontology, 42,* 44–49.

Robbins, M., & Francis, L. J. (2000). Religion, personality and well-being: The relationship between church attendance and purpose in life. *Journal of Research in Christian Education, 9*(2), 223–238.

Ryff, C. D. (1989). Happiness is everything, or is it? Explorations on the meaning of psychological well-being. *Journal of Personality and Social Psychology, 57,* 1069–1081.

Ryff, C. D., & Keyes, C. L. M. (1995). The structure of psychological well-being revisited. *Journal of Personality & Social Psychology, 69*(4), 719–727.

Ryff, C. D., & Singer, B. (1998). The contours of positive human health. *Psychological Inquiry, 9*(1), 1–28.

Ryff, C. D., Lee, Y. H., Essex, M. J., & Schmutte, P. S. (1994). My children and me: Midlife evaluations of grown children and of self. *Psychology and Aging, 9*(2), 195–205.

Ryff, C. D., Keyes, C. L. M., & Hughes, D. L. (2003). Status inequalities, perceived discrimination, and eudaimonic well-being: Do the challenges of minority life hone purpose and growth? *Journal of Health and Social Behavior, 44,* 275–291.

Schulenberg, S. (2004). A psychometric investigation of Logotherapy measures and the Outcome Questionnaire (OQ-45.2). *North American Journal of Psychology, 6*(3), 477–492.

Schulenberg, S., Gohm, C., & Anderson, C. (2006). The Meaning in Suffering Test (MIST): A unitary of multidimensional measure? *International Forum for Logotherapy, 29*(2), 103–106.

Schulenberg, S. E., Schnetzer, L. W., & Buchanan, E. M. (2011). The Purpose in Life test—Short form: Development and psychometric support. *Journal of Happiness Studies, 12,* 861–876.

Shek, D. T. L. (1993). The Chinese purpose-in-life test and psychological well-being in Chinese college students. *International Forum for Logotherapy, 16,* 35–42.

Shek, D. T. L. (1988). Reliability and factorial structure of the Chinese version of the Purpose in Life Questionnaire. *Journal of Clinical Psychology, 44*(3), 384–392.

Shek, D. T. L., Hong, E., & Cheung, M. Y. P. (1987). The Purpose in Life questionnaire in the Chinese context. *Journal of Psychology, 12,* 77–83.

Sink, C. A., van Keppel, J., & Purcell, M. (1998). Reliability estimates of the Purpose in Life and Seeking of Noetic Goals tests with rural and metropolitan area adolescents. *Perceptual and Motor Skills, 86,* 362.

Srole, L. (1956). Social integration and certain corollaries: An exploratory study. *American Sociological Review, 21,* 709–716.

Starck, P. L. (1983). Patients' perceptions of the meaning of suffering. *The International Forum for Logotherapy, 6,* 110–116.

Starck, P. L. (1985). *Guidelines—Meaning in suffering test.* Berkeley: Institute of Logotherapy Press.

Steger, M. F., & Kashdan, T. (2007). Stability and specificity of meaning in life and life satisfaction over one year. *Journal of Happiness Studies, 8,* 161–179.

Steger, M. F., Frazier, P., Oishi, S., & Kaler, M. (2006). The meaning in life questionnaire: Assessing the presence of and search for meaning in life. *Journal of Counseling Psychology, 53*(1), 80–93.

Steger, M. F., Kashdan, T., & Oishi, S. (2008). Being good by doing good: Daily eudaimonic activity and well-being. *Journal of Research in Personality, 42,* 22–42.

Stillman, T. F., Baumeister, R. F., Lambert, N. M., Crescioni, A. W., DeWall, C. N., & Fincham, F. D. (2009). Alone and without purpose: Life loses meaning following social exclusion. *Journal of Experimental Social Psychology, 45*(4), 686–694. doi:10.1016/j.jesp.2009.03.007.

Winston, R.B. Jr. (1988). Tools for assessing Students' Psychosocial development. *Georgia Journal of College Student Affairs,* 3(2), 15–20.

Winston, R. B. (1990). The student developmental task and lifestyle inventory: An approach to measuring students' psychosocial development. *Journal of College Student Development, 31*(2), 108–120.

Winston, R. B. Jr. & Miller, T. K. (1987). *Student Developmental Task and Lifestyle Inventory manual.* Athens, GA: Student Development Associates.

Winston, R. B., Miller, T. K., & Cooper, D. L. (1999). *Student developmental task and lifestyle assessment.* Athens: Student Development Associates.

Wong, P. T. P. (1998). Implicit theories of meaningful life and the development of the personal meaning profile. In P. T. P. Wong & P. S. Fry (Eds.), *The human quest for meaning: A handbook of psychological research and clinical applications* (pp. 111–140). Mahwah: Lawrence Erlbaum Associates Inc.

Yalom, I. (1980). *Existential psychotherapy.* New York: Basic Books.

Yeagar, D. S., & Bundick, M. J. (2009). The role of purposeful work goals in promoting meaning in life and school work during adolescence. *Journal of Adolescent Research, 24*(4), 423–452.

Chapter 3
The Role of Purpose in Optimal Human Functioning

As discussed in greater detail in Chap. 1 (Introduction and Definition), Viktor Frankl (1959), an Austrian Holocaust survivor, was the first psychiatrist to propose that having a purpose in life helped fend off negative states and promote well-being. According to Frankl, purposes are not given to people, instead they are discovered, and discovering a purpose helps individuals withstand the challenges they confront, both in dire conditions and in more typical daily life. Conversely, individuals who are either unwilling or unable to find a purpose are likely to experiencee "existential vacuum" or "existential neurosis," both of which refer to an intense sense of meaninglessness, manifest by an enduring subjective state of boredom, apathy, and emptiness.

Other researchers have extended and refined Frankl's theory of existential neurosis. For instance, Irvin Yalom (1980) considered meaning to be one of life's ultimate concerns, alongside death, isolation, and the loss of freedom, and he noted that individuals without meaning suffer significantly. As he put it, "the human being seems to require meaning. To live without meaning, goals, values, or ideals seems to provoke… considerable distress" (p. 422).

Similarly, Salvatore Maddi (1967) noted that existential neurosis features important cognitive, affective, and behavioral components. The cognitive component of existential neurosis is meaninglessness, or a chronic inability to believe that anything the individual is engaged in or could imagine being engaged in is important, useful, or interesting. The affective component is characterized by an overwhelming sense of blandness, boredom, and depression. Lastly, the behavioral component is evidenced by low activity level and a sense that activities are compelled rather than chosen. While all people are prone to moments of doubt and occasional passivity, individuals who suffer from existential neurosis experience these cognitive, affective, and behavioral features chronically.

According to Maddi (1967), certain individuals are more likely to experience existential neurosis than others. People who have an overly concrete and fragmentary sense of self are particularly vulnerable as they consider themselves nothing more than a "player of social roles and an embodiment of biological needs" (p. 315). These individuals may do fine for a time, experiencing only vague dissatisfaction and generalized anxiety; however, they often fall victim to existential

K. C. Bronk, *Purpose in Life*, DOI 10.1007/978-94-007-7491-9_3,

neurosis when they encounter stressors that require them to see the limitations of their biological selves, such as when they are forced to confront their own mortality. They are also at risk if they experience circumstances that call into question their system of social roles. For example, in times of economic or social upheaval it may become impossible to obtain the usual rewards for fulfilling certain social roles. This can occur when economic recessions hit and the breadwinner loses his or her job. In these instances, individuals who conceive of themselves merely as fillers of social roles are particularly likely to suffer existential neurosis.

While Frankl's ideas were primarily theoretical in nature, other researchers have conducted studies that offer broad, empirical support for many of them. A series of studies, for example, sought to determine if there was an empirical basis for his existential theory, which suggests that boredom is the result of purposelessness, and results consistently suggest there is. For example, a cluster of studies confirm that boredom is distinct from depression and anxiety (Fahlman et al. 2009), that individuals in a high purpose state report less boredom than individuals in a low purpose state (Fahlman et al. 2009), that chronically bored individuals typically lack a life purpose (Drob and Bernard 1988), and that turning away from or leaving meaningful life projects leads to a sense of being stuck in a chronic state of boredom (Bargdill 2000). Results of a longitudinal study of meaning and boredom conclude that these two factors likely share a bidirectional, causal relationship (Fahlman et al. 2009), whereby a sense of meaninglessness causes boredom and vice versa. Taken together these studies offer strong support for the inverse relationship between purpose and boredom.

Further, empirical studies also conclude that purposelessness not only contributes to existential neurosis, but also to other negative outcomes and psychological states. For example, studies have determined that purposelessness is related to psychopathology (Kish and Moody 1989), as Frankl asserted, and to antisocial behavior (Shek et al. 1994). Individuals without a purpose in life are more likely to dwell on problems, blame others, and report high levels of anger and negative affect (Sappington and Kelly 1995). A series of studies examined the relationship among purpose, hope, and depression and concluded that purpose is positively related to hope and inversely related to depression. Mascaro and Rosen (2005) concluded that explicit meaning, which is defined as having a philosophy or framework that provides a sense of coherence and purpose, and implicit meaning, which is defined as a sense of personal meaningfulness, were related to increased levels of state and trait hope and decreased levels of depression. Results were similar among a clinical population (Debats 1996). Other studies have similarly concluded that purpose is inversely related to loneliness (Paloutzian and Ellison 1982), psychosocial problems (Ho et al. 2010), general anxiety, and depression (Bigler et al. 2001).

Also consistent with Frankl's theory, purposelessness has been found to be higher among individuals suffering from mental illness. For example, a series of studies have shown that psychiatric patients score lower on purpose than more typical individuals do (Chaudary and Sharma 1976; Crumbaugh and Maholick 1967; Gonsalevz and Gon 1983). Researches have concluded on the basis of their work with psychiatric patients that a lack of purpose in life may be a cause of the development of some conventional psychopathological syndromes (Gonsalvez and Gon 1983). However, given the cross-sectional rather than longitudinal nature of these studies, the causal nature of this relationship cannot be confirmed (Moomal 1999).

Along these same lines, empirical research also finds that purposelessness, or having few meaningful reasons to live, is associated with a lack of hope and suicide ideation (Dixon et al. 1991; Edwards and Holden 2001; Heisel and Flett 2004; Kinnier et al. 1994; Harlow et al. 1986). Heisel and Flett (2004) examined the role of purpose and life satisfaction in protecting against suicide ideation among a clinical sample, and they concluded that low purpose and life satisfaction scores accounted for significant additional variability in suicide ideation scores above and beyond that accounted for by negative psychological factors, such as neuroticism, depression, and social hopelessness. Studies also find that purpose and meaning mediate the relationship between life satisfaction and suicide ideation, and moderate the relationship between depression and suicide ideation (Heisel and Flett 2004). Similarly, meaninglessness has been found to mediate the relationship between depression and self-derogation (Morojele and Brook 2004; Harlow et al. 1986).

Meaninglessness and purposelessness predict not only suicide ideation, but also overt forms of suicide behavior. One study found that students without strong reasons for living were more likely to give up attempts to resolve stress and hopelessness and were more likely to move from suicide ideation to suicide behavior (Bonner and Rich 1987). Similarly, a lack of a sense of coherence, including meaninglessness, appears to serve as a precursor to suicide (Mohler-Kuo et al. 2006; Kinnier et al. 1994; Petrie and Brook 1992). These stark findings underscore the importance of focusing on purpose and meaning from a clinical as well as a research perspective.

In sum, a growing body of empirical work demonstrates strong support for the existence of existential neurosis. As Frankl predicted, numerous studies confirm that meaninglessness and purposelessness strongly predict boredom (Fahlman et al. 2009; Drob and Bernard 1988; Bargdill 2000), suicide ideation (Mohler-Kuo et al. 2006; Petrie and Brook 1992; Kinnier et al. 1994), and other negative psychological states (Harlow et al. 1986; Kish and Moody 1989).

Stress

Another negative psychological state related to purpose is stress. However, the relationship between purpose and stress is not as straightforward as the relationship between purposelessness and other negative indicators of psychological health. Researchers have argued that working to preserve and promote one's purpose in life can actually increase stress levels, at least in the short term. Lazarus and DeLongis (1983), for example, argued that sources of personal meaning influence the stress and coping process as events in life that challenge important commitments, such as purposes, are likely to be apprised as threats, and as such are likely to increase one's perceived stress level. In this way, pursuing purpose may increase stress, especially when individuals feel their purposeful aims are being threatened (Zika and Chamberlain 1992).

Another way purpose has been linked to stress is through engagement in personally meaningful, but stressful, activities. The act of leading a purposeful life and engaging in purposeful activities may itself be stressful and may lead to more negative affect (Hughes 2006). For example, parenting and care giving represent activities that can be incredibly stressful, but that can also be tremendously meaningful. Parents (Umberson and Gove 1989) and caregivers (Marks et al. 2002) report lower levels of positive affect than non-parents and non-caregivers, but at the same time, they report higher levels of purpose. It is evident, then, that pursuing some kinds of purposes may result is heightened stress levels.

On the other hand, a relatively large body of research concludes that purpose and stress are inversely related. For example, research finds that maintaining a meaningful purpose in life is associated with positive coping (Kass et al. 1991) and decreased stress levels (Ishida and Okada 2006; Stevens et al. 1987), including decreased acculturative stress (Pan et al. 2008). Additionally, a recent empirical study determined that a transcendent sense of meaning, which shares with purpose a commitment to promoting aims beyond-the-self, moderated the effects of stress, depression, and mental health problems among Chinese college students (Hong 2008), and a similar study determined that American college students who deemed their lives meaningful were less likely to report feeling stressed (Steger and Frazier 2005). Still another study concluded that meaning in life served as a protective factor for Chinese students studying abroad in an English speaking country (Pan et al. 2008). Lower levels of acculturative stress were associated with higher levels of meaning in life, which predicted higher levels of life satisfaction. Taken together then, we can conclude that in some instances purpose and stress are inversely related.

At first glance, findings regarding the relationship between purpose and stress appear to be contradictory: individuals who pursue purpose are likely to be more stressed as a result of their purposeful engagement, but at the same time, individuals with purpose are likely to cope better and report lower stress levels overall. It seems likely that timing plays a role here. In the short run, individuals with purpose may experience greater stress levels than individuals without purpose, as they inevitably confront challenges associated with pursuing their personally meaningful aspirations. However, in the long run, they may experience less stress knowing that these challenges are in service of a larger goal. Three complementary theories attempt to further clarify this complex relationship between purpose and stress.

The first theory suggests that individuals with purpose are likely to be exposed to more stressors, but they are better equipped than individuals without purposes to handle them. While leading a life of purpose may be stressful, the coherence that purpose provides bolsters an individual's ability to bounce back from challenges, and as such purposeful individuals are better equipped to deal with purpose-related stress and other stressors. Empirical research identifies purpose as a protective factor that contributes to resiliency (Benard 1991; Masten and Reed 2002), Antonovsky (1979, 1987) argues that individuals who possess a clear sense of coherence, or a belief that their lives make sense and that they are manageable and meaningful, believe they can meet life's demands and overcome its obstacles. Put another way, as a result of pursuing personally meaningful aspirations, individuals with purpose may indeed encounter additional stressors, but because of the strong sense of coherence in their lives, they are able to bounce back from these challenges more easily than they would if they lacked purpose.

A related theory suggests that like resilient individuals, people who demonstrate hardiness are also better equipped to handle the stressors associated with leading a life of purpose. Hardiness is associated with a strong sense of control, challenge, and, similar to purpose, commitment. It is evident among individuals who are able to remain calm and function at high levels in potentially stressful situations (Kobasa 1979). The three dispositions of commitment, control, and challenge lead hardy individuals to engage in activities and events rather than to stand passively by, to experience a sense of control over the things that happen in their lives, and to believe that obstacles and difficulties are a normal part of life and that they can offer valuable opportunities for growth. Accordingly, commitment to overcoming obstacles coupled with a sense of efficacy that obstacles are surmountable allows hardy individuals, similar to purposeful individuals, to conquer potentially stressful situations.

These resiliency perspectives suggest that purposeful individuals evaluate potentially stressful situations the same way more typical individuals do, but that they are better equipped than other people to handle stress. Other scholars see it differently.

A second theory of stress and purpose suggests that purposeful individuals actually assess potentially stressful situations differently than more typical individuals. In this perspective, the sense of direction that results from leading a life of purpose helps individuals manage stress because they view potentially stressful situations through a particular lens. "A focus on these larger purposes of life creates long range contexts that connect the past with the future and take us way beyond the experience of our present selves" (Hughes 2006, p. 623). In other words, leading a life of purpose orients individuals to the long-term rather than the short-term, and potentially short-term stressors are not deemed to be as stressful when viewed through a long range lens. Further, pursuing purpose yields a sense of unity to people's worldviews (Lazarus and De Longis 1983; Zika and Chamberlain 1992), and this far-horizon focus allows them to interpret potentially stressful situations as more manageable in nature.

Along these same lines, a leading scholar of youth purpose, William Damon (2008, 2011), argues that people, in particular youth, may not experience work in pursuit of purpose as stressful, even when it is difficult. Instead, purposeful youth are capable of working hard and pushing themselves as long as they know what they are working for. "The biggest problem growing up today is not actually stress; it's meaninglessness" (Damon 2011). In short, challenges that lack meaning—not hard work—cause stress. Damon argues that working hard for something that one does not believe in or for something that one does not choose is not only counterproductive, but also unsustainable. On the other hand, working hard for something that one does believe in—even when doing so could be considered stressful by others—is not likely to be experienced as stressful at all. Instead the experience can unleash tremendous energy, creativity, exhilaration, and a deep sense of satisfaction with efforts and accomplishments. In this way, people with strong commitments to purposes do not experience potentially stressful challenges as stress inducing. Instead, they view them as meaningful challenges to be overcome in the pursuit of a larger aim.

The third way that purpose can protect individuals from stress is through supportive social networks. A small body of empirical research suggests that having a purpose in life serves to connect purposeful individuals to others, and this too can help them handle stress more effectively. Pursing a purpose may "enhance the quality of life by motivating people's involvement in activities that promote social integration and the quality of social relationships" (Hughes 2006, p. 611). In essence, individuals who lead lives of purpose are more likely to encounter positive social networks that can help them effectively cope with the additional stressors they are likely to encounter. A longitudinal study found that this was indeed the case for a small sample of intensely purposeful youth (Bronk 2008). As a result of pursuing purposes, these youth encountered supportive peer and mentoring relationships that fostered their healthy development and enhanced their overall sense of well-being. Along the same lines, research finds that high purpose scores predict sociability (Pearson and Sheffield 1974) and social participation (Doerries 1970; Yarnell 1971). Research on the hardy personality provides additional evidence for the relationship between purpose and social support. Ganellen and Blaney (1984) found that the challenge and commitment dimensions of the hardy profile, the latter of which shares important features with purpose, strongly correlate with social support. "Hardy individuals tend to be more active in seeking out social support, especially in stressful situations. Alternatively, other studies suggest that a lack of purpose predicts an array of psychosocial problems that may serve to isolate individuals and sever these potentially protective connections. For example, meaninglessness is associated with avoiding social situations (e.g. alienation) and having a powerful fear of humiliation (e.g. social maladjustment) (Ho et al. 2010). Other studies similarly conclude that meaninglessness may negatively influence relational connectedness, resulting in social disturbances and even social rejection (Cacioppo et al. 2005).

In sum, pursuing a life of purpose may expose people to new sources of stress, but purposeful individuals tend to be hardy and resilient, and consequently, they are better prepared to bounce back from the potentially stressful challenges and setbacks they encounter. It may also be the case that purposeful individuals who find themselves working for something they believe in do not interpret challenging circumstances as stressful at all. They may do this because they maintain a long-range focus and because they evaluate these challenges as worthwhile and unavoidable in pursuit of a larger, personally meaningful aim. Additionally, in the course of pursuing purpose, individuals are likely to come into contact with others who share their interests and commitments, and this can result in the formation of a positive developmental context and a supportive social network that not only fosters the growth of purpose directly, by providing information and resources, but also indirectly, by helping individuals effectively manage the potential stressors associated with leading a life of purpose. These emerging theories on the relationship between purpose and stress are not mutually exclusive; it seems likely that under different circumstances each helps explain why it is that individuals who encounter extra stressors associated with purpose are less likely to succumb to the negative effects of stress. However, additional research is needed to assess the relationship among these theories and to explore the circumstances under which each best explains this complex relationship.

Coping and Substance Abuse

Another way individuals with purpose manage to handle stress effectively has to do with the coping mechanisms they utilize. Compared to individuals with low meaning scores, individuals with high meaning scores report less avoidance coping (e.g. ignoring the problem and hoping it will go away) and more emotion-focused coping (e.g. changing one's emotional reaction to the stressor) (Edwards and Holden 2001). Other research finds that high purpose scores predict more mature defense mechanisms and more mature coping strategies (Whitty 2003).

Drug and alcohol use represent particularly negative coping mechanisms, and empirical studies consistently find that purpose and substance abuse are inversely related (Coleman et al. 1986; Padelford 1974; Sayles 1994; Schlesinger et al. 1990). Further, researchers have determined that meaninglessness mediates the relationship between uncontrollable stress and substance use among adolescents (Newcomb and Harlow 1986). Purpose is similarly negatively related to other potentially dangerous, addictive behaviors. A recent study, for example, found that nicotine and food addictions were significantly negatively related to the presence of purpose among Japanese college students (Okasaka et al. 2008).

Purposelessness is clearly related to dependence, but the promising news is that discovering a purpose appears to be associated with recovery from addiction. Participants in an in-patient alcohol and drug treatment program reported purpose in life scores that were significantly lower than average before treatment but that were within the normal range after treatment (Waisberg and Porter 1994). Additionally, higher purpose scores at the end of treatment predicted improved relationships, better health, and less alcohol and drug use at a follow-up (Waisberg and Porter 1994). A similar study found that overcoming drug addition predicted higher purpose scores (Noblejas de la Flor 1997), and a study of Alcoholics Anonymous members concluded that purpose positively correlated with length of sobriety (Carroll 1993). Finally, a third study concluded that drug addicts were less likely than non-addicts to report a well-defined sense of meaning in life (Coleman et al. 1986).

In addition to helping to establish the relationship between purposelessness and substance abuse, Newcomb and Harlow (1986) have offered a useful explanation of the mechanism behind the association. This team of researchers argues that among adolescents, anyway, "stressful life events lead to a perceived loss of control, which leads to meaninglessness, which in turn leads to substance abuse" (p. 565). In this model, the association between stress and substance abuse is mediated by meaning and purpose. Though alcohol and drug use among adolescents is multiply determined, data exist to support this chain of relationships. Interestingly, however, results vary somewhat based on gender; confronted by a lack of purpose, women are apt to turn to substance abuse while men are apt to consider suicide (Newcomb and Harlow 1986).

It has been well established that purpose is associated with resiliency (Benard 1991), hardiness (Kobasa 1979), and effective coping mechanisms (Edwards and Holden 2001; Whitty 2003). It is also evident that purpose buffers against negative states such as boredom (Bargdill 2000; Drob and Bernard 1987), anxiety (Bigler et al. 2001), and depression (Bigler et al. 2001). However, each of these orientations to purpose assumes a background of danger, deficit, and challenge in people's lives, all of which must be overcome by the development of a personal resiliency borne of protective factors, such as purpose. A growing body of more contemporary research reveals that beyond merely helping individuals avoid and manage negative states, pursing a purpose in life can actually promote positive states, including psychological and even physical well-being.

Psychological and Physical Well-being

As discussed in greater detail in Chap. 1 (Introduction and Definition), pursuing a life purpose is a central component of many leading theories of optimal human development. Having a life purpose represents a key component of Ryff's (Ryff and Singer 2008) conception of eudaimonia, which emphasizes the goal of self-actualization; it signifies an important path to well-being in Seligman's (2011) conception of flourishing; and it characterizes a transcendent virtue in Peterson and Seligman's (2004) character strengths model. In addition to being a significant component of healthy adult growth (Seligman 2011; Ryff and Singer 1998b; Boyle et al. 2009), having purpose is also critical part of positive youth development (Benson 2006; Damon 2004, 2008; Lerner et al. 2005; Shek 1992). Benson (2006) considered it an important internal developmental asset, and Lerner and colleagues (Lerner et al. 2005) see contribution, which is closely related to purpose, as a desirable outcome of healthy growth. In some conceptions of well-being, purpose is seen as an indicator of thriving (Benson 2006; Bundick et al. 2010; Gillham et al. 2011), in others as an outcome (Lerner et al. 2005), and in still others as a defining feature of it (Ryff and Singer 1998a; Seligman 2011), but regardless of its particular role, it is clear that purpose is strongly associated with optimal development.

Psychological well-being encompasses a variety of positive psychological states, and purpose has been associated with many of these, including subjective well-being (Gillham et al. 2011; Seligman 2002; Zika and Chamberlain 1987), self-esteem (Bigler et al. 2001; Paloutzian and Ellison 1982; Scannell et al. 2002; Schlesinger et al. 1990), and quality of existence (Hughes 2006; Shek 1992). Purpose has also been found to predict two related aspects of psychological well-being: happiness

(French and Joseph 1999; Lewis et al. 1997), and positive affect (King et al. 2006; Noblejas de la Flor 1997). However, here the relationship is less straightforward. As already discussed, purpose and positive affect are not always positively correlated. Some pursuits of purpose, such as parenting (Umberson and Gove 1989), caregiving (Marks et al. 2002), and likely others, perhaps volunteering, teaching, and counseling, can be difficult, tiresome, and trying, but in the long run, they can also be incredibly meaningful. Happiness represents a mood or a fleeting emotion, and at times the pursuit of purpose, at least certain kinds of purpose, is likely to be a decidedly unhappy experience. Parents must tell their children no, and caregivers must comfort loved ones who are hurting. Accordingly, it is important to distinguish, as Seligman (2011) does, between happiness and flourishing. While only some forms of purpose appear to be associated with happiness and positive affect, most appear to be elements of optimal well-being.

This conclusion is supported by a large body of research that consistently concludes that purpose and psychological well-being are positively associated. Zika and Chamberlain (1992) found that studies using a variety of measures of purpose, including the Purpose in Life Test (PIL; Crumbaugh 1968; Crumbaugh and Maholick 1964), the Sense of Coherence measure (SOC; Antonovsky 1983, 1987), and the Life Regard Index (LRI; Battista and Almond 1973; Debats et al. 1995) all yielded significant, positive correlations between purpose and psychological well-being. Interestingly, these studies included both midlife and later adult participants, and the results were the same regardless of the participants' age. The researchers conclude that the association between purpose and psychological well-being is strong, and that over time the source of purpose may change, but its relation to psychological well-being does not.

Pursuing purpose is also associated with increased levels of life satisfaction (Gillham et al. 2011; Peterson et al. 2005), though the relationship varies whether one considers the presence of or the search for purpose. Empirical studies conclude that having a purpose in life predicts higher life satisfaction scores for adolescents (Bronk et al. 2009), emerging adults (Bronk et al. 2009; Steger et al. 2006), and midlife adults (Bronk et al. 2009), but searching for a purpose in life only predicts higher life satisfaction scores for adolescents and emerging adults (Bronk et al. 2009). Searching for a purpose does not predict increased life satisfaction for midlife adults. These findings make sense in light of societal expectations. In most Western cultures it is a normative experience for adolescents and emerging adults to be actively involved in the search for purpose, and therefore it makes sense that the search at these stages is accompanied by higher ratings of life satisfaction, but by adulthood individuals are expected to have found a purpose for their lives. Those individuals who are still searching report, not surprisingly, feeling less satisfied with their lives. This research has been confined to western individuals. Future studies should investigate the relationship between the presence of purpose and the search for purpose among individuals at different stages of life in different cultures to see if the same pattern of results emerges.

Not only is the presence of purpose significantly associated with life satisfaction, but it also appears to be an important component of the good life. Among college and community samples, perceptions of a good life typically include the sense that one's life is meaningful (King and Napa 1998). Interestingly, this study concluded that moral goodness is an even more significant indicator of a good life than wealth.

Purpose has also been called an ego strength (Markstrom et al. 1997; Shek 1992) and a character strength and virtue (Peterson and Seligman 2004). As an ego strength, purpose is defined as having the courage to envision and pursue personally meaningful aims (Erikson 1964). Maintaining a life purpose allows adolescents to imagine who they hope to become and what they hope to accomplish in their lives (Bronk 2011; Markstrom et al. 1997). As a character strength, purpose is categorized alongside the virtues of spirituality, religiousity, and faith, and features a focus on the "transcendent (nonphysical) dimension of life" (Peterson and Seligman 2004, p. 600). Common to both of these conceptions of purpose is a focus on the positive role this construct plays in healthy human development. Interestingly, empirical studies find that the positive role of purpose is largely related to the subjective sense that one's life is meaningful rather than the presence of life goals (Shek 1992). In other words, *feeling* that one's life is purposeful is at least as important in conveying the benefits of purpose as is *acting* on one's aspirations. That said, both affective and cognitive aspects of life meaning serve as important indicators of positive mental health (Shek 1992).

By now it should be clear that leading a life of purpose is critical to positive mental health. A relatively large body of empirical research supports this claim. However, a small but growing body of research is beginning to shed light on the role purpose plays not only in fostering psychological health, but also in promoting positive physical health. Ryff and Singer (1998b) argue that psychological and physical health are closely aligned, and given that purpose is consistently associated with psychological well-being, it is not surprising to find that it is also increasingly associated with physical well-being.

A fever, chills, and a headache may serve as useful signs of illness, but what are the corresponding signs of health? Often times we consider health to be the absence of illness (e.g. no fever, no chills, and no headache), but according to Ryff and her colleagues, being well means more than just *not* being ill (Ryff and Singer 1998a). It means being able to strive toward one's full potential, and to do that individuals need to possess the six attributes assessed by Ryff's Scales of Psychological Well-being, which are discussed in greater detail in Chap. 2 (Measuring Purpose). Briefly, the six attributes include self-acceptance, positive relations with others, autonomy, environmental mastery, personal growth, and purpose in life (Ryff 1989). In this conception of health, purpose represents not just an indicator of well-being, but a defining feature of it (Ryff and Singer 1998a). An individual with a strong sense of purpose "has goals in life and a sense of directedness; feels there is meaning to present and past life; holds beliefs that give life purpose; (and) has aims and objectives for living" (Ryff and Singer 2008, p. 25).

Many of the studies that explore the relationship between purpose and health rely on the Scales of Psychological Well-being purpose subscale (Ryff and Keyes 1995). One such study determined that individuals with high purpose scores report a variety of improved markers of health (Ryff et al. 2004). For example, older women with higher levels of purpose tend to show flatter diurnal slopes of daily salivary cortisol than those with lower levels of purpose. Specifically, older women who were purposefully engaged in life started the day with lower cortisol levels that stayed lower throughout the day compared with women who reported lower purpose scores. This means that purposeful engagement is significantly related to lower stress hormone levels, and this is important since high stress hormone levels are associated with a wide range of negative health effects.

This same study also determined that purpose was linked to pro-inflammatory cytokines, specifically the soluble receptor for IL-6, that high levels of purposeful engagement among older women was positively associated with lower levels of inflammation response, and that higher purpose scores were linked to improved cardiovascular and metabolic markers (Ryff et al. 2004). Older women with higher purpose scores had lower levels of glycosylated hemoglobin, lower waist-hip ratios, and lower total/HDL cholesterol ratios, and weighed less than those with lower purpose scores. Higher levels of purposeful engagement were also associated with higher levels of HDL, the good cholesterol. All of these relationships were modest, but the overall trend clearly suggests that purpose is associated not only with psychological well-being, but also with important indicators of physical health as well. These findings are particularly noteworthy because individuals who scored high in hedonic well-being (as opposed to eudaimonic well-being, which features purpose) did not report significant health improvements. In other words, it seems likely that purpose, rather than pleasure or happiness, contributes to these physical benefits.

A longitudinal study using this same measure of purpose concluded that rates of Alzheimer's Disease and mild cognitive impairment were significantly lower among individuals with higher purpose scores (Boyle et al. 2010). In fact, a person with a particularly high score (90th percentile) on Ryff's purpose in life subscale was 2.4 times more likely to remain free of Alzheimer's Disease than a person with a particularly low purpose score (10th percentile). Interestingly, this association did not vary along demographic lines and persisted even after the addition of terms for depressive symptoms, neuroticism, social network size, and the number of chronic medical conditions.

Perhaps not surprisingly, given that purpose appears to be associated with a wide range of positive health outcomes, another study using Ryff and colleagues measure (Ryff and Keyes 1995) concluded that higher life purpose scores were also associated with a reduced risk of all-cause mortality among community dwelling older adults (Boyle et al. 2009; Krause 2009).

Studies using different measures have come to similar conclusions regarding the healthful correlates of leading a life of purpose. For example, a study using the Life Attitude Profile (LAP; Reker and Peacock 1981; Reker et al. 1987) concluded that a lack of purpose was associated with perceived psychological and physical discomforts (Reker et al. 1987), and a study employing the Inventory of Positive Psychological Attitudes (IPPA; Kass et al. 1991) determined that individuals who reported high levels of purpose, life satisfaction, and self-confidence suffered less chronic pain (Kass et al. 1991). Similarly, another study of pain management, using Antonovsky's Sense of Coherence measure (SOC; 1983, 1987) concluded that meaningfulness predicted self-reports of decreased pain at a six month follow up (Petrie and Azariah 1990). Lastly, Melnechuk (1988) summarized a body of literature based on a range of measures that related positive feelings, religious beliefs, and expressions of various goals and hopes, which at least potentially overlap with purposes, to the regression of cancers and other autoimmune disorders.

Taken together, the results of these studies indicate that purposelessness is consistently associated with pathological outcomes, and that purpose is related to positive physical and psychological outcomes. Interestingly, purpose appears to correlate more strongly and more consistently with positive psychological outcomes than purposelessness does with pathological outcomes.

Most of the studies of purpose and physical health are correlational in nature. Consequently, it is impossible to know if pursuing purpose leads to better health or if having better health leads individuals to discover purpose, or if a third factor, such as social connectedness, is responsible for both higher rates of purpose and improved physical health. Each of these routes seems plausible, and additional studies designed to tease out the direction and nature of the relationship are warranted.

Purpose and Health Behaviors

In addition to predicting physical health, purpose is also significantly associated with wide variety of positive health behaviors. For example, research converges to suggest that purposeful individuals are more likely to be prosocially engaged than their non-purposeful peers (Damon et al. 2003), and higher scores on the Purpose in Life test (PIL; Crumbaugh 1968; Crumbaugh and Maholick 1967) correlate with increased levels of altruism (Shek et al. 1994; Noblejas de la Flor 1997). Similarly, higher generativity scores, a construct that shares with purpose a commitment to contributing to matters beyond-the-self, are associated with increased levels of social activity and political activism (McAdams 2001).

Further, a series of studies of exposure to violence and victimization among African American adolescents living in public housing reveals that purpose can buffer youth from potentially negative environmental influences. DuRant and colleagues discovered that purpose scores, as measured by the Purpose in Life test (PIL; Crumbaugh 1968; Crumbaugh and Maholick 1964), inversely related to the number of sexual partners adolescents' reported having in the past three months (DuRant et al. 1995) and to the self-reported use of violence (DuRant et al. 1994). The authors concluded that having a life purpose serves as a protective factor that can help shield young people from the potentially negative effects of growing up in distressed communities.

In sum, a growing body of research suggests that purpose is a critical component of well-being and positive mental health. Less well understood, however, is *how* purpose facilitates both physical and psychological well-being. Ryff and Singer (1998a) have proposed three potential paths through which purpose may facilitate well-being. The first theory suggests that purpose is a defining feature of positive mental health; having good health *means* having purpose. Second, Ryff and Singer have argued that the central components of positive mental health are consequential for physical health. In other words, things are happening inside the body during the experience of purposeful living that are advantageous to one's health. For example, it may be the case that certain areas of the brain are activated during purposeful engagement that likewise support physical health. And, third, "it is the reciprocal, interactive nature of these mental/physical, mind/body connections that are at the heart of understanding positive human health" (Ryff and Singer 1998a). In other words, individuals who are mentally well are also likely to be physically well as the two systems impact and are impacted by one another. Which of these mechanisms offers the best description of the relationship between psychological and physical health has yet to be determined.

Regardless of the precise nature, the strong and consistent relationship between purpose and psychological and physical health is noteworthy. Both cognitive dimensions of purpose (personally meaningful beliefs and goals) (Ho et al. 2010) and affective dimensions (subjective feelings that one's life is meaningful) (Scannell et al. 2002) of meaning significantly relate to indicators of well-being (Moomal 1999), and the relationship between purpose and psychological health is evident in studies employing a wide range of measures of purpose and closely related constructs (e.g. PIL; DuRant et al. 1995, 1994; Crumbaugh and Maholick 1969; Zika and Chamberlain 1992; Moomal 1999; SOC; Zika and Chamberlain 1992; Antonovsky 1987; LRI; Zika and Chamberlain 1992; Scannell et al. 2002, MLQ; Steger and Frazier 2005; IPPA; Kass et al. 1991, Scales of Psychological Well-being; Ryff and Singer 1998a). Studies have determined that purposelessness correlates with negative outcomes (e.g. Bargdill 2000; Bigler et al. 2001; Drob and Bernard 1987; Ishida and Okada 2006; Stevens et al. 1987) and that the presence of purpose correlates with positive outcomes for children (Benson 2006), adolescents (Lerner et al. 2005; Damon 2008; Newcomb and Harlow 1986; Markstrom et al. 1997; Ho et al. 2010; Shek et al.1994; Shek 1992; Gillham et al. 2011), college students (King and Napa 1998; Steger and Frazier 2005; Hong 2008; Debats et al. 1993; Moomal 1999), young adults (DuRant et al. 1995; DuRant et al. 1994), midlife adults (Bronk et al. 2009; Scannell et al. 2002), and later adults (Ryff and Singer 2008). These findings strongly suggest that the pursuit of purpose is a healthy activity across the lifespan.

Purpose also appears to benefit individuals from different ethnic backgrounds, including individuals from Japan (e.g. Okasaka et al. 2008), China (e.g. Hong 2008; Ho et al. 2010; Shek et al. 1994; Shek 1992), South Africa (e.g. Morojele and Brook 2004; Moomal 1999), Australia (e.g. Scannell et al. 2002), and America (e.g. Steger and Frazier 2005; Damon 2008). Clinical (e.g. Dixon et al. 1991; Heisel and Flett 2004), community (King and Napa 1998; Scannell et al. 2002; Debats et al. 1993), and college samples (Steger and Frazier 2005; Bronk et al. 2009; Moomal 1999) all appear to benefit from having a sense of purpose and meaning in life, and purpose appears to be at least moderately correlated with nearly every component of well-being (Zika and Chamberlain 1992). Though we cannot discern causation from these results, we can conclude that individuals who lack purpose and meaning in life are likely to show detrimental effects in a wide range of aspects of psychological functioning, and that individuals with a sense of purpose and meaning in life are poised to thrive.

The strong and consistent relationship between purpose and positive psychological outcomes raises at least one concern that needs to be addressed. Correlations this pervasive suggest some level of confound between the constructs; it is possible that measures of purpose and psychological well-being lack sufficient discriminant validity (Zika and Chamberlain 1992). However, while there may be some overlap between these two constructs, leading a life of purpose does appear to uniquely contribute to well-being. This is consistently evident since none of the studies discussed found a one-to-one relationship between psychological well-being and purpose. It is also clear that purpose and meaning are not synonymous with positive affect. While some purposes correlate with positive affect (King et al. 2006; Noblejas de la Flor 1997), others do not. Hughes (2006) highlighted the distinction between at least some purposes and affect by citing a series of studies in which the two variables are independent of one another. While purpose may not be synonymous with well-being, the strong correlations do point to at least some level of overlap. This suggests as Ryff and Singer (1998a) propose, that purpose may be a defining feature of well-being.

Other Positive Correlates of Purpose

Not only is purpose associated with positive psychological and physical health, but emerging research finds it is also related to other aspects of well-being. For instance, having a purpose in life appears to support academic achievement and to contribute to professional satisfaction.

As discussed in greater detail in Chap. 2 (Measuring Purpose), Chickering and Reisser (1993) devised a model of college student growth that features seven vectors of healthy college student development. Each vector represents a series of developmental tasks that college students must accomplish. Developing purpose, one of the critical developmental tasks in this model, refers to determining why one is attending college, what one hopes to accomplish through his or her education, and what one hopes to achieve professionally and personally. In other words, Chickering and Reisser see developing purpose as a critical part of a successful college experience.

Perhaps one reason purpose is associated with more successful educational experiences is because students who have a clear vision of what they are working for are likely to not only be more motivated, but are also likely to enjoy the challenges associated with working hard in school. To this end, a recent study investigated the relationship between the nature of adolescents' work goals and their ratings of subjective well-being (Yeager and Bundick 2009). Self-reported work goals varied along two dimensions: whom students felt they should be working for and what students said they hoped to accomplish with their jobs. In terms of whom they were working for, students were categorized as maintaining work goals either focused on serving themselves or others, and with regards to what they hoped to accomplish, students' professional aims could either be intrinsic to the nature of the job or extrinsic to it. *Purposeful work goals* represented professional aims that were intended to serve others through the intrinsic nature of the job. For example, an individual who wanted to become a nurse to help make sick people more comfortable was said to have a purposeful work goal. Only 30 % of adolescents espoused purposeful work goals, but those who did reported higher levels of purpose in general and said that studying and doing homework was more meaningful compared to youth with other kinds of professional aims.

Another way that purpose is likely related to academic achievement is through its relationship with grit. Not surprisingly, individuals who demonstrate grit, or the tendency to stick with things until they are mastered, perform better in school (Duckworth et al. 2007). Grit is associated with purpose (Hill, Burrow, and Bronk, under review) and individuals with purpose are more likely to report increases in grit over time than individuals without purpose (Hill et al. under review). This is important given that grittiness without purpose may lack direction, but with purpose, it can promote dedication to the academic goals required to support personally meaningful, long-term aims.

Perhaps as a result of being grittier, individuals with purpose report feeling better equipped to handle academic challenges. In fact, an empirical study revealed that purpose was significantly related to three different measures of self-efficacy (DeWitz et al. 2009), including the College Self-Efficacy Inventory (Solberg et al. 1993), the Scale of Perceived Social Self-Efficacy (Smith and Betz 2000), and the General Self-Efficacy Subscale of the Self Efficacy Scale (Sherer et al. 1982). We cannot discern from these correlational studies which comes first, purpose or self-efficacy; empirical studies are needed to test the causal relationship. If, however, results conclude that self-efficacy leads to purpose, then creating interventions designed to boost students' sense of self-efficacy may positively influence students' subjective sense of purpose and improve college student retention.

Given that purpose is associated with achievement motivation and academic self-efficacy, it is not surprising to find that an emerging line of inquiry also suggests that fostering purpose may lead to higher levels of academic achievement. A recent study concluded that as levels of purpose and internal locus of control increased, so too did grade point averages, at least among low-income youth (Pizzolato et al. 2011). While not suggestive of a causal relationship, research on "sparks," a common indicator of purpose, similarly reveals that youth who are able to identify the activities that inspire them and who have support for pursing those interests also report higher grade point averages (Benson 2008). Together these studies make a strong case for directly assessing, among a diverse sample, the relationship between purpose and academic achievement; the results of such a study would be compelling.

Having a purpose in life influences not only school experiences, but also professional experiences. College students with purpose report greater clarity regarding their future occupational plans than youth without purpose (Tryon and Radzin

1972). This makes sense given that one of the main functions of purpose is to orient individuals in a particular direction or in pursuit of a specific aim. Of course, a purpose does not need to take the form or a job, but whether it does or not, purpose is likely to, at least indirectly, influence career choices. Individuals who find purpose in caring for their families, for instance, might consider jobs that allow them to spend considerable time at home with their children, and individuals who find purpose in serving God, may seek professional avenues that align with their religious convictions. In other cases, purposes can directly influence career choices. For instance, an individual committed to caring for animals may become a veterinarian, while an individual who finds purpose in helping children may become a social worker. Individuals who are purposefully engaged through work not only derive increased levels of meaning from their jobs but also report enjoying their jobs more than individuals who do not find their work meaningful (Bonebright et al. 2000). They also show fewer signs of workaholism (Bonebright et al. 2000).

Meaningful careers, often referred to as "callings" or "vocations" (Damon 2008; Weiler and Schoonover 2001), can be elusive. Consequently, a cottage industry designed to help students (e.g. Dik et al. 2011; Kosine et al. 2008) and adults (e.g. Leider 1997) select careers that advance their purposes has emerged. One such "purpose-centered approach" to career development provides a model that school counselors can use to aid students in developing a sense of purpose in their career search through employing strengths-based practices (Kosine et al. 2008). The authors present five key elements that reinforce the growth of purpose, including identity, self-efficacy, metacognition, culture, and service. Each of these areas is used as a focal point to help identify ways students can recognize and rely on their strengths as they devise meaningful career plans. For instance, with regards to identity students are encouraged to explore who they are and how that image intersects with who they hope to become and what they hope to do professionally, and with regards to self-efficacy, students are exposed to jobs that make use of their personal strengths and rely on their academic interests. A career counseling program based on these principles was recently implemented at a middle school, and students who participated in the program developed a stronger sense of direction in their career choices, a clearer recognition of their interests, strengths and weaknesses, and a greater level of preparedness for the future as compared to youth who did not participate in the program (Dik et al. 2011). Another such program features five steps that individuals should follow to discover fulfilling careers (Weiler and Schoonover 2001). These steps include changing old mindsets about work, contracting for renewal, finding one's calling, making it happen, and staying the course.

It is interesting to note that, like these two approaches, many career counseling programs assume that individuals have a purpose before they begin working. While this may be the case for some individuals, it is likely not the case for all. Instead, some individuals find themselves doing jobs that over time take become personally significant. Interestingly, a study of young purpose exemplars revealed that engaging in activities that subsequently became meaningful was more common than seeking out meaningful activities (Bronk 2012).

A full discussion of the career counseling for purpose literature, some of which is empirically based and some of which is based on personal opinion or experience, is beyond the scope of this book, but the fact that such a niche exists underscores the pervasiveness of the purpose construct in career planning.

Finally, other aspects of optimal development relevant to purpose will be discussed later in this book. For example, research finds that purpose is a key component of healthy identity development, and healthy identity formation is essential to psychological health and well-being (Erikson 1963). The close relationship between purpose and identity development is elaborated upon in Chap. 4 (Purpose across the Lifespan). Beyond identity, purpose has also been found to contribute to well-being through religion. A full discussion of the relationship among well-being, religiosity, and purpose can be found in Chap. 6 (Inspiring Types of Purposes in Life). Lastly, purpose is also related to a wide range of positive values and virtues including hope (Bronk et al. 2009), humility (Bronk 2008), anti-materialism (Crandall and Rasmussen 1975; Maddi 1967), and optimism (Ho et al. 2010), and these findings are discussed in greater detail in Chap. 7 (The Experience of Purpose among Diverse Groups).

In sum, purpose clearly plays a central role in optimal well-being, and though it appears to be advantageous to pursue purpose at any stage of life, the way in which individuals find and pursue meaningful aspirations changes across the lifespan. The following chapter synthesizes research on the developmental trajectory of purpose.

References

Antonovsky, A. (1979). *Health, stress, and coping*. San Francisco: Jossey Bass.

Antonovsky, A. (1983). The sense of coherence: Development of a research instrument. *Newsletter and Research Reports, 1,* 1–11.

Antonovsky, A. (1987). *Unraveling the mystery of health*. San Francisco: Jossey Bass.

Bargdill, R. W. (2000). The study of boredom. *Journal of Phenomenological Psychology, 31,* 188–219.

Battista, J., & Almond, R. (1973). The development of meaning in life. *Psychiatry, 36,* 409–427.

Benard, B. (1991). *Fostering resiliency in kids: Protective factors in the family, school, and community*. Portland: Northwest Regional Educational Laboratory.

Benson, P. L. (2006). *All kids are our kids: What communities must do to raise caring and responsible children and adolescents* (2nd ed.) San Francisco: Jossey-Bass.

Benson, P. L. (2008). *Sparks: How parents can help ignite the hidden strengths of teenagers*. San Francisco: Jossey Bass.

Bigler, M., Neimeyer, G. J., & Brown, E. (2001). The divided self revisited: Effects of self-concept clarity and self-concept differentiation on psychological adjustment. *Journal of Social and Clinical Psychology, 20,* 396–415.

Bonebright, C. A., Clay, D. L., & Ankenmann, R. D. (2000). The relationship of workaholism with work-life conflict, life satisfaction, and purpose in life. *Journal of Counseling Psychology, 47,* 469–477.

Bonner, R., & Rich, A. (1987). Toward a predictive model of suicide ideation and behavior: Some preliminary data in college students. *Suicide and Life Threatening Behavior, 17,* 50–63.

Boyle, P. A., Barnes, L. L., Buchman, A. S., & Bennett, D. A. (2009). Purpose in life is associated with mortality among community-dwelling older persons. *Psychosomatic medicine, 71*(5), 574–9.

Boyle, P. A., Barnes, L. L., Buchman, A. S., & Bennett, D. A. (2010). Effect of a Purpose in life on risk of incident Alzheimer Disease and mild cognitive impairment in community-dwelling older persons. *Archives of general psychiatry, 67*(3), 304–310. doi: 10.1001/archgenpsychiatry.2009.208.

Bronk, K. C. (2008). Humility among adolescent purpose exemplars. *Journal of Research on Character Education, 6*(1), 35–51.

Bronk, K. C., Hill, P. L., Lapsley, D. K., Talib, T., & Finch, W. H. (2009). Purpose, hope, and life satisfaction in three age groups. *Journal of positive psychology, 4*(6), 500–510.

Bundick, M. J., Yeager, D. S., King, P. E., & Damon, W. (2010). Thriving across the lifespan. In R. M. Lerner, M. E. Lamb, A. M. Freund, & W. F. Overton (Eds.), *Handbook of life- span development, Vol. 1: Cognition, Biology and Methods* (pp. 882–923). Hoboken: Wiley.

Bronk, K. C. (2011). Portraits of purpose: The role of purpose in identity formation. *New Directions for Youth Development, 132,* 31–44.

Bronk, K. C. (2012). A grounded theory of Youth purpose. *Journal of Adolescent Research, 27,* 78–109.

Cacioppo, J. T., Hawklwy, L. C., Rickett, E. M., & Masi, C. M. (2005). Sociality, spirituality, and meaning making: Chicago health, aging, and social relations study. *Review of General Psychology, 9,* 143–155.

Carroll, S. (1993, May). Spirituality and purpose in life in alcoholism recovery. *Journal of Studies on Alcohol, 54*(3), 297–301.

Chaudary, P. N., & Sharma, V. (1976). Existential frustration and mental illness: A comparative study of purpose in life in psychiatric patients and normals. *Indian Journal of Clinical Psychology, 3,* 171–174.

Chickering, A. W., & Reisser, L. (1993). *Education and identity (2nd ed.).* San Francisco: Jossey-Bass.

Coleman, S., Kaplan, J., & Downing, R. (1986). Life cycle and loss: The spiritual vacuum of heroin addiction. *Family Process, 25,* 5–23.

Crandall, J. E., & Rasmussen, R. D. (1975). Purpose in life as related to specific values. *Journal of Clinical Psychology, 31,* 483–485.

Crumbaugh, J. C. (1968). Cross-validation of Purpose in Life test based on Frankl's concepts. *Journal of Individual Psychology, 24,* 74–81.

Crumbaugh, J. C., & Maholick, L. T. (1964). An experimental study in existentialism: The psychometic approach to Frankl's concept of noogenic neurosis. *Journal of Clinical Psychology, 20,* 200–207.

Crumbaugh, J. C., & Maholick, L. T. (1967). An experimental study in existentialism: The psychometric approach to Frankl's concept of noogenic neurosis. In V. E. Frankl (Ed.), *Psychotherapy and existentialism* (pp. 183–197). New York: Washington Square Press.

Crumbaugh, J. C., & Maholick, L. T. (1969). *Manual of Instructions for the Purpose in Life test. Munster.* IN: Psychometric Affiliates.

Damon, W. (Jan. (2004). What is positive youth development? *The Annals of the American Academy of Political and Social Science, 591,* 13–24.

Damon, W. (2008). *The path to purpose: Helping our children find their calling in life.* San Francisco: Jossey Bass.

Damon, W. (Nov. 18, 2011). Getting off the treadmill: Finding purpose, by Terry Lobdell. *Palo Alto Daily News* (37–48).

Damon, W., Menon, J., Bronk, K. C. (2003). The development of purpose during adolescence. *Applied Developmental Science, 7*(3), 119–128.

Debats, D. L. (1996). Meaning in life: Clinical relevance and predictive power. *British Journal of Clinical Psychology, 35*(4), 503–516.

Debats, D. L., Drost, J., & Hansen, P. (1995). Experiences of meaning in life: a combined qualitative and quantitative approach. *British Journal of Psychology, 86,* 359–375.

Debats, D. L., van der Lubbe, P. M., Wezerman, F. R. A. (1993). On the psychometric properties of the Life Regard Index (LRI): A measure of meaningful life: An evaluation in three independent samples based on the Dutch version. *Personality and Individual Differences, 14,* 337–345.

DeWitz, S. J., Woolsey, M. L., & Walsh, B. W. (2009). College student retention: An exploration of the relationship between self-efficacy beliefs and purpose in life among college students. *Journal of College Student Development, 50*(1), 19–34.

Dik, B. J., Steger, M. F., Gibson, A., & Peisner, W. (2011). Make Your Work Matter: Development and pilot evaluations of a purpose-centered career education intervention. *New Directions for Youth Development, 132,* 59–73.

Dixon, W., Heppner, P., & Anderson, W. (1991). Problem-solving appraisal, stress, hopelessness, and suicide ideation in a college population. *Journal of Counseling Psychology, 38,* 51–56.

Doerries, L. E. (1970). Purpose in life and social participation. *Journal of Individual Psychology, 26,* 50–53.

Drob, S. L., & Bernard, H. S. (1988). The bored patient: A developmental existential perspective. *Psychotherapy Patient, 3*(3–4), 63–73.

Duckworth, A. L., Peterson, C., Matthews, M. D., & Kelly, D. R. (2007). Grit: Perseverance and passion for long-term goals. *Journal of Personality and Social Psychology, 92*(6), 1087–1101.

DuRant, R. H., Cadenhead, C., Pendergast, R. A., Slavens, G., & Linder, C. W. (1994). Factors associated with the use of violence among urban Black adolescents. *American Journal of Public Health, 84*(4), 612–617.

DuRant, R. H., Getts, A., Cadenhead, C., Emans, S. J., & Woods, E. R. (1995). Exposure to violence and victimization and depression, hopelessness, and purpose in life among adolescents living in and around public-housing. *Journal of Development and Behavioral Pediatrics, 16*(4), 233–237.

Edwards, M. J., & Holden, R. R. (2001). Coping, meaning in life, and suicidal manifestations: Examining gender differences. *Journal of Clinical Psychology, 57,* 1517–1534.

Erikson, E. H. (1963). *Childhood and society*. New York: W. W. Norton.

Erikson, E. H. (1964). *Insight and responsibility*. New York: W.W. Norton.

Fahlman, S. A., Merce, K. B., Gaskovski, P., Eastwood, A. E., & Eastwood, J. D. (2009). Does a lack of life meaning cause boredom? Results from psychometric, longitudinal and experimental analyses. *Journal of Social and Clinical Psychology, 28*(3), 307–340.

Frankl, V. E. (1959). *Man's search for meaning: An introduction to logotherapy*. Boston: Beacon Press.

French, S., & Joseph, S. (1999). Religiosity and its association with happiness, purpose in life, and self-actualization. *Mental Health, Religion, & Culture, 2,* 117–120.

Ganellen, R. J., & Blaney, P. H. (1984). Hardiness and social support as moderators of the effects of life stress. *Journal of Personality and Social Psychology, 47,* 156–163.

Gillham, J., Adams-Deutsch, Z., Werner, J., Reivich, K., Coulter-Heindl, V., Linkins, M., Winder, B., Peterson, C., Park, N., Abenavoli, R., Contero, A., & Seligman, M. E. P. (2011). Character strengths predict subjective well-being during adolescence. *Journal of Positive Psychology, 6*(1), 31–44. doi: 10.1080/17439760.2010.536773.

Gonsalvez, G. J., & Gon, M. (1983). A comparative study of purpose in life in psychopathological and normal groups. *Indian Journal of Clinical Psychology, 10,* 211–218.

Harlow, L. L., Newcomb, M. D., & Bentler, P. M. (1986). Depression, self-derogation, substance use, and suicide ideation: Lack of purpose in life as a meditational factor. *Journal of Clinical Psychology, 42*(1), 5–21.

Heisel, M. J., & Flett, G. L. (2004). Purpose in life, satisfaction with life, and suicide ideation in a clinical sample. *Journal of Psychopathology and Behavioral Assessment, 26*(2), 127–135.

Hill, P. L., Burrow, A. L., & Bronk, K. C. (under review). Grit during a college semester: The role of purpose.

Ho, M. Y., Cheung, F. M., & Cheung, S. F. (2010). The role of meaning in life and optimism in promoting well-being. *Personality and individual differences, 48*(5), 658–663.

Hong, L. (2008, June). College stress and psychological well-being: Self-transcendence meaning of life as a moderator. *College Student Journal, 42*(2), 531–541.

Hughes, M. (2006). Affect, meaning and quality of life. *Social Forces, 85*(2), 611–629.
Ishida, R., & Okada, M. (2006). Effects of a firm purpose in life on anxiety and sympathetic nervous activity caused by emotional stress: Assessment by psycho-physiological method. *Stress and Health: Journal of the International Society for the Investigation of Stress, 22*(4), 275–281.
Kass, J. D., Friedman, R., Leserman, J., Caudill, M., Zuttermeister, P. C., & Benson, H. (1991). An inventory of positive psychological attitudes with potential relevance to health outcomes: Validation and preliminary testing. *Behavioral Medicine, 17*(3), 121–129.
King, L. A., Hicks, J. A., & Krull, J., & Del Gaiso, A. K. (2006). Positive affect and the experience of meaning in life. *Journal of Personality and Social Psychology, 90,* 179–196.
King, L. A., & Napa, C. K. (1998). What makes a life good? *Journal of Personality and Social Psychology, 75,* 156–165.
Kinnier, R., Metha, A. T., Keim, J. S., Okey, J. L., Adler-Tabia, R., Berry, M. A., & Mulvenon, S. W. (1994). Depression, meaninglessness, and substance abuse in "normal" and hospitalized adolescents. *Journal of Alcohol and Drug Education, 39*(2), 101–111.
Kish, G. B., & Moody, D. R. (1989). Psychopathology and life purposes. *International Forum for Logotherapy, 12*(1), 40–45.
Kobasa, S. C. (1979). Stressful life events, personality, and health: An inquiry into hardiness. *Journal of Personality and Social Psychology, 37,* 1–11.
Kosine, N. R., Steger, M. F., & Duncan, S. (2008). Purpose-centered career development: A strengths-based approach to finding meaning and purpose in careers. *Professional School Counseling, 12*(2), 133–136.
Krause, N. (2009). Meaning in life and mortality. *The Journals of Gerontology Series B: Psychological Sciences and Social Sciences, 64B*(4), 517–527. doi: 10.1093/geronb/gbp047
Lazarus, R. S., & DeLongis, A. (1983). Psychological stress and coping in aging. *American Psychologist, 38,* 245.
Leider, R. (1997). *The power of purpose: Creating meaning in your life and work.* San Francisco: Berrett-Koehler Publishers.
Lerner, R. M., Lerner, J. V. L., Almerigi, J. B., Theokas, C., Phelps, E., Gestsdottir, S., Naudeau, S., Jelicic, H., Alberts, A., Ma, L., Smith, L. M., Bobek, D. L., Richman-Raphael, D., Simpson, I., Christiansen, E. D., & von Eye, A. (2005). Positive youth development, participation in community youth development programs, and community contributions of fifth-grade adolescents: Findings from the First wave of the 4-H study of positive youth development. *Journal of Early Adolescence, 25*(1), 17–71.
Lewis, C. A., Lanigan, C., Joseph, S., & de Fockert, J. (1997). Religiosity and happiness: No evidence for an association among undergraduates. *Personality and Individual Differences, 22,* 119–121.
Maddi, S. R. (1967). The existential neurosis. *Journal of Abnormal Psychology, 72,* 311–325.
Marks, N. F., Lambert, J. D., & Choi, H. (2002). Transitions to caregiving, gender, and psychological well-being: A prospective U. S. national study. *Journal of Marriage and Family, 64,* 657–67.
Markstrom, C. A., Sabino, V. M., Turner, B. J., & Berman, R. C. (1997). The psychosocial inventory of ego strengths: Development and validation of a new Eriksonian measure. *Journal of Youth and Adolescence, 26*(6), 705–732.
Mascaro, N., & Rosen, D. H. (2005). Existential meaning's role in the enhancement of hope and prevention of depressive symptoms. *Journal of Personality, 73*(4), 985–1013.
Masten, A. S., & Reed, M. G. J. (2002). Resilience in development. In C. R. Snyder, & S. J. Lopez (Eds.), *Handbook of positive psychology* (pp. 74–88). New York: Oxford University Press.
McAdams, D. P. (2001). Generativity in midlife. In M. Lackman (Ed.), *Handbook of midlife development* (pp. 395–443). New York: Wiley.
Melnechuk, T. (1988). Emotions, brain, immunity, and health: A review. In M. Clynes, & J. Panksepp (Eds.), *Emotions and psychopathology* (pp. 181–247). New York: Plenum.
Mohler-Kuo, M., Wydler, H., Zellweger, U., & Gutzwiller, F. (2006). Differences in health status and health behavior among Swiss adults between 1993–2003. *Swiss Medical Weekly, 136*(29–30), 464–72.

Moomal, Z. (1999). The relationship between meaning life and mental well-being. *South African Journal of Psychology, 29*(1), 42–50.

Morojele, N. K., & Brook, J. S. (2004). Sociodemographic, sociocultural, and individual predictors of reported feelings meaninglessness among South African adolescents. *Psychological Reports, 95*(3), 1271–1278.

Newcomb, M. D., & Harlow, L. L. (1986). Life events and substance use among adolescents: Mediating effects of perceived loss of control and meaninglessness in life. *Journal of Personality and Social Psychology, 51*(3), 564–577.

Noblejas de la Flor, M. A. (1997). Meaning levels and drug abuse therapy: An empirical study. *International Forum for Logotherapy, 20*(1), 46–51.

Okasaka, Y., Nobuaki, M., Nakatani, Y., & Fujisawa, K. (2008). Correlation between addictive behaviors and mental health in university students. *Psychiatry and Clinical Neuroscience, 62,* 84–92.

Padelford, B. L. (1974). Relationship between drug involvement and purpose in life. *Journal of Clinical Psychology, 30,* 303–305.

Paloutzian, R. F., & Ellison, C. W. (1982). Loneliness, spiritual well-being, and quality of life. In L. A. Peplau, & D. Perlman (Eds.), *Loneliness: A Sourcebook of Current Theory, Research, and Therapy*. New York: Wiley.

Pan, J. Y., Wong, D. F. K., Joubert, L., Chan, C. L. W. (2008). The protective function of meaning of life on life satisfaction among Chinese students in Australia and Hong Kong: A cross-cultural comparative study. *Journal of American College Health, 57*(2), 221–231.

Pearson, P. R., & Sheffield, B. F. (1974). Purpose-in-life and the Eysenck Personality Inventory. *Journal of Clinical Psychology, 30*(4), 562–564.

Peterson, C., Parks, N. S., & Seligman, M. E. P. (2005). Orientations to happiness and life satisfaction: The full life versus the empty life. *Journal of Happiness Studies, 6,* 25–41.

Peterson, C., & Seligman, M. E. P. (2004). *Character strengths and virtues: A handbook and classification*. New York: Oxford University Press.

Petrie, K., & Azariah, R. (1990). Health-promoting variables as predictors of response to a brief pain management program. *Clinical Journal of Pain, 6*(1), 43–46.

Petrie, K., & Brook, K. (1992). Sense of coherence, self-esteem, depression, and hopelessness as correlates of reattempting suicide. *British Journal of Clinical Psychology, 31,* 293–300.

Pizzolato, J. E., Brown, E. L., & Kanny, M. A. (2011). Purpose plus: Supporting youth purpose, control, and academic achievement. *New Directions for Youth Development, 132,* 75–88.

Reker, G. T., & Peacock, E. J. (1981). The life attitude profile (LAP): A multidimensional instrument for assessing attitudes toward life. *Canadian Journal of Behavioural Science, 13,* 64–73.

Reker, G. T., Peacock, E. J., & Wong, P. T. P. (1987). Meaning and purpose in life and well-being: A life-span perspective. *Journal of Gerontology, 42*(1), 44–49.

Reker, G. T., & Wong, P. T. P. (1988). Aging as an individual process: Toward a theory of personal meaning. In J. E. Birren, & V. L. Bengston (Eds.), *Emergent theories of aging* (pp. 214–246). New York: Springer.

Ryff, C. D. (1989). Happiness is everything, or is it? Explorations on the meaning of psychological well-being. *Journal of Personality and Social Psychology, 57,* 1069–1081.

Ryff, C. D., & Keyes, C. L. M. (1995). The structure of psychological well-being revisited. *Journal of Personality and Social Psychology, 69*(4), 719–727.

Ryff, C. D., & Singer, B. (1998a). The role of purpose in life and personal growth in positive human health. In P. T. P. Wong (Ed.), *The human quest for meaning: A handbook of psychological research and applications (2nd ed.)* (pp. 213–235). New York: Routledge.

Ryff, C. D., & Singer, B. (1998b). The contours of positive human health. *Psychological Inquiry, 9*(1), 1–28.

Ryff, C. D., & Singer, B. (2008). Know thyself and become what you are: A eudaimonic approach to psychological well-being. *Journal of Happiness Studies, 9,* 13–39.

Ryff, C. D., Singer, B., & Love, G. D. (2004). Positive health: Connecting well-being with biology. *Philosophical Transactions: Biological Sciences, 359,* 1383–1394.

Sappington, A. A., & Kelly, P. J. (1995). Self perceived anger problems in college students. *International Forum for Logotherapy, 18,* 74–82.

Sayles, M. L. (1994). Adolescents' purpose in life and engagement in risky behaviors: Differences by gender and ethnicity. (Doctoral dissertation, University of North Carolina at Greensboro, 1994). *Dissertation Abstracts International, 55,* 09A2727.

Scannell, E. D., Allen, F. C. L., & Burton, J. (2002). Meaning in life and positive and negative well-being. *North American Journal of Psychology, 4*(1), 93–111.

Schlesinger, S., Susman, M., & Koenigsberg, J. (1990). Self-esteem and purpose in life: A comparative study of women alcoholics. *Journal of Alcohol and Drug Education, 36,* 127–141.

Seligman, M. E. P. (2002). *Authentic happiness: Using the new positive psychology to realize your potential for lasting fulfillment.* New York: Free Press.

Seligman, M. E. P. (2011). *Flourishing: New York: A visionary new understanding of happiness and well-being.* New York: Free Press.

Shek, D. (1992). Meaning in life and psychological well-being: An empirical study using the Chinese version of the purpose in life questionnaire. *Journal of Genetic Psychology, 153,* 185–190.

Shek, D. T. L., Ma, H. K., & Cheung, P. C. (1994). Meaning in life and adolescent antisocial and prosocial behavior in a Chinese context. *Psychologia, 37,* 211–218.

Sherer, M., Maddux, J. E., Mercandante, B., Prentice-Dunn, S., Jacobs, B., & Rogers, R. W. (1982). The Self-Efficacy Scale: Construction and validation. *Psychological Reports, 51,* 663–671.

Smith, H., & Betz, N. E. (2000). Development and evaluation of a measure of social self-efficacy in college students. *Journal of Career Assessment, 8,* 282–302.

Solberg, V. S., O'Brien, K., Villareal, P., Kennel, R., & Davis, B. J. (1993). Self-efficacy and Hispanic college students: Validation of the college self-efficacy instrument. *Hispanic Journal of Behavioral Sciences*, 15, 80–95.

Steger, M. F. & Frazier, P. (2005). Meaning in life: One link in the chain from religiousness to well-being. *Journal of Counseling Psychology, 52*(4), 574–582.

Steger, M. F., Frazier, P., Oishi, S., & Kaler, M. (2006). The Meaning in Life Questionnaire: Assessing the presence of and search for meaning in life. *Journal of Counseling Psychology, 53,* 80–93.

Stevens, M. J., Pfost, K. S., & Wessels, A. B. (1987). The relationship of purpose in life to coping strategies and time since the death of a significant other. *Journal of Counseling and Development, 65,* 424–426.

Tryon, W., & Radzin, A. (1972). Purpose-in-life as a function of ego resiliency, dogmatism, and biographical variables. *Journal of Clinical Psychology, 28,* 544–545.

Umberson, D., & Gove, W. (1989). Parenthood and psychological well-being: Theory, measurement, and stage in the life course. *Journal of Family Issues, 10,* 440–462.

Waisberg, J., & Porter, J. (1994). Purpose in life and outcomes of treatment for alcohol dependence. *British Journal of Clinical Psychology, 33,* 49–63.

Weiler, N. W., & Schoonover, S. C. (2001). *Your soul at work: Five steps to a more fulfilling career and life*. Mahwah: Hidden Spring.

Whitty, M. T. (2003). Coping and defending: Age differences in maturity of defense mechanisms and coping strategies. *Aging and Mental Health, 7,* 123–132.

Yalom, I. (1980). *Existential psychotherapy*. New York: Basic Books.

Yarnell, T. D. (1971). Purpose in life test: Further correlates. *Journal of Clinical Psychology, 27,* 76–79.

Yeager, D. S., & Bundick, M. (2009). The role of purposeful life goals in promoting meaning in life and schoolwork during adolescence. *Journal of Adolescent Research, 24*(4), 423–452.

Zika, S., & Chamberlain, K. (1987). Relation of hassles and personality to subjective well-being. *Journal of Personality and Social Psychology, 53,* 155–162.

Zika, S., & Chamberlain, K. (1992). On the relation between meaning in life and psychological well-being. *British Journal of Psychology, 83,* 133–145.

Chapter 4
Purpose across the Lifespan

For some, identifying, committing to, and pursuing purpose is a life long process. Theoretical and empirical research explores purpose in childhood (Erikson 1968, 1980), adolescence (e.g. Damon 2008; Francis and Evans 1996; Martinez and Dukes 1997; Yeagar and Bundick 2009), emerging adulthood (e.g. Bronk et al. 2009; McLean and Pratt 2006), midlife (e.g. Crumbaugh and Maholick 1967; Ryff et al. 2003; Ryff and Singer 2008), later adulthood (Laufer et al. 1981; Greenfield and Marks 2004; Pinquart 2002), and across the lifespan (Baum and Stewart 1990; Fegg et al. 2007). Historically, purpose was primarily considered a feature of adulthood (Frankl 1959; Ryff 1989). However, more recently, given the growing body of empirical evidence that young people often commit to meaningful purposes (Bronk et al. 2009; Bronk et al. 2010; Damon 2008; Moran 2009) and given the close relationship between the growth of purpose and identity formation (Bronk 2011; Burrow and Hill 2011; Damon 2008; Hill and Burrow 2012), the construct has more commonly been associated with adolescence and emerging adulthood.

While people can develop a purpose any time after late childhood, research suggests that purposeful activity often begins during childhood, becomes intentional and meaningful during adolescence and emerging adulthood, and evolves throughout midlife and later adulthood. This chapter synthesizes research on purpose across the lifespan.

Childhood

Little empirical work focuses on purpose during childhood. This is likely because children are cognitively constrained (VanDyke and Elias 2007). Unable to engage in the planning and hypothetical-deductive reasoning required to identify and commit to purpose, children are unlikely to seriously consider personally meaningful, long range aspirations. However, experiences in childhood can set the stage for the subsequent development of purpose. For example, research suggests that individuals who report more positive experiences in childhood are more likely to report

K. C. Bronk, *Purpose in Life*, DOI 10.1007/978-94-007-7491-9_4,

purposes later in life (Ishida and Okada 2006), especially in emerging adulthood (Mariano and Vaillant 2012).

Along these same lines, a longitudinal study with a small sample of young people with intense commitments to various purposes concluded that while these youth did not commit to purposes prior to adolescence, they did engage in potentially purposeful activities during childhood (Bronk 2012). This study consisted of a dozen young people who participated in in-depth interviews about their aspirations three times over a five-year period, spanning later adolescence and early emerging adulthood (Bronk 2011, 2012; Damon 2008). In interviews, each of the participants reported that they first became involved in activities that later evolved into purposes during the early elementary school years. For instance, a young man in his twenties, committed to sharing jazz music with a broader audience, traced the roots of his commitment to elementary school, when he began playing the piano. Similarly, a young man committed to raising money to supply clean drinking water to people in need reported learning about and becoming active in the cause in first grade when his teacher talked to his class about the need for safe water sources in developing countries. Another youth, who would later dedicate her life to serving God, began learning about her faith when her Dad and stepmother first took her to church in second grade. Each of the individuals in the exemplar sample was able to trace his or her purpose to an activity that began during childhood. This suggests that for at least some young people, purposeful interests take root relatively early in the lifespan.

Findings from this longitudinal study also suggest that extracurricular activities and opportunities during childhood may foster the development of purpose (Bronk 2012). Had the musician lived in an area where he lacked easy access to musical instruction, or had the religious exemplar never been taken to church, it is possible that neither of these youth would have developed purposes. This suggests that early involvement may contribute to subsequent purpose development.

Beyond the opportunities afforded by a particular locale, it is also evident that the nature of one's hometown can influences the types of purposes to which young people aspire (Bronk 2012). For example, in the study of purpose exemplars, a young woman reflected on her environmental aspirations:

> I guess because I live out here, really. Everything that is out here is what we use. We live off of our own water under our own land…. I think that's a big part of why environmental work is such a big deal, because I live out in the country. I live in the environment.

Another exemplar, committed to curbing gun violence, noted that growing up in an area where bank shoot-outs and killings occurred during his childhood influenced his commitment to gun control. The other exemplars similarly cited access to people, places, and opportunities associated with where they grew up as central to their subsequent commitments to various life purposes.

These findings are based on a small sample of intensely committed young people's retrospective accounts of early experiences, and they should be considered in light of these limitations. However, it can be concluded that childhood *can* play a key role in the later development of purpose, and this has important implications for how parents, teachers, and adults concerned with the well-being of young people should attempt to foster purpose. While adults should never try to be the driving force behind a young person's purpose (Damon 2008), it is important for them to introduce young people to a variety of potentially purposeful activities during childhood as doing so may provide young people with opportunities to discover aspirations that they may find personally meaningful and to which they may be well suited (Bronk 2012). A fuller discussion of the ways in which purpose can intentionally be fostered follows in Chap. 5 (Origins of and Supports for Purpose).

Adolescence and Emerging Adulthood

While children may engage in potentially purposeful activities, it is not until adolescence and emerging adulthood that individuals are likely to seriously consider and intentionally commit to a purpose. Committing to a purpose appears to support positive youth development in a variety of important ways. As discussed in greater detail in the preceding chapter, committing to a purpose predicts happiness (French and Joseph 1999; Lewis et al. 1997), hope (Bronk et al. 2009), life satisfaction (Bronk et al. 2009; Gillham et al. 2011; Peterson et al. 2005) and flourishing (Seligman 2011). Accordingly, a life purpose is a critical developmental asset for youth (Benson 2006; Damon 2008) and a key component of their psychological well-being (Zika and Chamberlain 1992). Further, pursing purpose can contribute to a more meaningful academic experience (Yeagar and Bundick 2009) and can help connect youth with like-minded peers and supportive mentors (Bronk 2012). Another important way that leading a life of purpose benefits youth is through its association with healthy identity development (Bronk 2012; Burrow et al. 2010; Damon 2008; Erikson 1968, 1980; Fry 1998).

Identity Identity formation is central to healthy growth across the lifespan, but it takes special prominence during adolescence and emerging adulthood (Arnett 2000; Erikson 1968). In Erikson's time the search for identity corresponded closely with adolescence; today it often happens later (Schwartz et al. 2005; Schwartz and Montgomery 2002). In late-modern societies, the realities and experiences of childhood and adolescence have been increasingly distinct from the realities and experiences of adulthood (Côté 2000; Côté and Allahar 1996; Côté and Levine 2002; Schwartz 2007). Consequently, the gulf between these two stages has widened, leading to the recognition of a new stage of life: emerging adulthood (Arnett 2000). So, while Erikson associated identity with the adolescent life stage, researchers today increasingly associate it with emerging adulthood (Arnett 2000; Schwartz 2007). Because the development of identity and the related search for purpose span the adolescent and emerging adult periods, these two life stages are discussed together here.

During identity development, young people experiment with different roles and try-out various personalities to determine who they are and where they fit in with the broader world (Erikson 1968, 1980). Adolescents and emerging adults typically consider, among other issues, their professional plans, their religious and political beliefs, and the type of romantic partner they hope to find. They are also likely to reflect on the centrality or personal significance of each of these issues.

The search for identity represents a critical developmental task. Young people who fail to adequately sort out issues of identity emerge from this stage of life with a negative identity or a diffuse sense of self (Erikson 1968, 1980), while youth who successfully navigate this task emerge with a coherent, stable, and flexible sense of who they are and an increased capacity for well-being. According to Erikson (1980), the successful completion of identity development leads to fidelity, or a commitment to a particular set of values and beliefs. This far horizon commitment can form the contours of a life purpose. Accordingly, in developing a lasting sense of who they are, youth often simultaneously reflect on the roles they hope to hold and the personally meaningful goals they hope to accomplish. Fidelity is evident when young people start working toward personally meaningful roles and long-term aims. Some have argued that fidelity represents an important, alternate perspective on a contemporary rite of passage (Markstrom et al. 1998). In this view, figuring out who one is and what one hopes to accomplish represents an important marker on the path to adulthood.

Not only do purpose and identity develop at roughly the same time, but they also share a focus on personally meaningful beliefs and aims. However, despite their concomitant appearance in the lifespan and their shared focus, they describe distinct constructs. Identity refers to *who* one is likely to become while purpose refers to *what* one hopes to achieve (Bronk 2011).

Additionally, while all youth eventually explore and/or commit to an identity, only a relatively small proportion of young people discover their purpose. Empirical studies, employing different measures of purpose and different samples of youth, consistently conclude that only about 25 % of young people commit to a clear purpose in life (Bronk et al. 2010; Damon 2008; Francis 2000; Moran 2009). Rates of purpose are slightly lower among adolescents (20 %) and somewhat higher among emerging adults (30 %; Bronk et al. 2010; Damon 2008; Moran 2009). While youth with a clear sense of purpose are relatively rare, youth who demonstrate some signs of purpose are more common. Roughly 55 % of young people show some signs of purpose, and they can be categorized into one of two groups: those who hold self-oriented life goals and those who are dreamers (Damon 2008). Individuals who hold self-oriented life goals are actively engaged in working toward an aim that is personally meaningful, but it is a long-term aim that is purely self-serving. For instance, they may aim to maximize their wealth, happiness, power, or personal sense of security. Because their aspirations lack a beyond-the-self focus, these individuals lack a clear sense of purpose. On the other hand, dreamers are individuals who have identified a personally meaningful, long-term, beyond-the-self aim, but who have failed to do anything about it. Because they have not begun working on their goals and because they lack clear plans on how to get started, they also fail to meet the full definition of purpose. Finally, the remaining 20 % of youth show no signs of purpose at all. Individuals in this cluster are unable to articulate personally meaningful, long-term aims of any sort.

Erikson (1968) believed that under ideal circumstances purpose and identity developed together, and researchers have recently begun to investigate the interconnected relationship between these two constructs. A series of empirical studies suggests that individuals tend to commit to identities and purposes at roughly the same time. For example, a recent study concluded that increased commitments in purpose development corresponded to increased commitments in identity development (Hill and Burrow 2012), and a study of turning point life narratives found that young people who had begun identity exploration by age nineteen were more likely to discuss meaning-making experiences in their life narratives at age twenty-three (McLean and Pratt 2006). Adolescents' purpose scores have also been shown to positively predict identity formation scores (Schwartz 2007).

Along these same lines, a recent study examined identity development according to Marcia's (1966) theories of "individual styles of coping" (p. 558). Marcia called these styles "identity statuses," and assigned individuals to them based on their level of identity commitment (high or low) and identity exploration (high or low). As such, four statuses exist: achievement (high commitment; high exploration); moratorium (low commitment; high exploration); foreclosure (high commitment; low exploration); and diffusion (low commitment; low exploration). Burrow et al. (2010) found that the growth of adolescent purpose appears to follow existing formulations of identity development. A hierarchical clustering strategy identified four distinct purpose profiles, including *achieved, foreclosed, uncommitted,* and *diffused,* that largely corresponded with Marcia's (1966) identity statuses. For instance, youth categorized as identity achieved were also categorized as purpose achieved (high purpose commitment and high purpose exploration), and youth categorized as identity foreclosed were also categorized as purpose foreclosed (high in purpose commitment and low in purpose exploration). In sum, the growth of purpose appears to correspond closely to the process of identity formation.

Conclusions from a similar study offer additional support for the correspondence between identity and purpose development. This study concluded that individuals in the identity achievement status tended to report a greater sense of future purpose than individuals in the identity moratorium status (Côté and Levine 1982). Individuals in the identity diffuse and identity foreclosure statuses did not significantly differ from one another or from individuals in the other two statuses with regards to their purpose scores. Another study of 12,000 adolescents found that ethnic identity development coincided with purpose development, and that increased levels of ethnic identity development corresponded with increased evidence of purpose (Martinez and Dukes 1997). Further, a study exploring the relationship among identity statuses, purpose, and well-being, determined that higher diffuse/avoidant identity statuses correlated with lower well-being scores overall and lower purpose scores in particular (Vleioras and Bosma 2005). Taken together, these studies offer strong empirical support for Erikson's (1968, 1980) proposition that identity and purpose can progress together; as individuals develop a clearer sense of who they hope to become, they are also likely to develop a clearer sense of what they hope to accomplish.

Perhaps one reason these constructs develop at roughly the same time is because growth around purpose spurs growth around identity, and vice versa. Put another way, these constructs may reinforce one another (Hill and Burrow 2012). This theory is supported by results of a longitudinal study that reveal that for those young people who discover purpose, the process of doing so can facilitate identity formation (Bronk 2011). As a result of being actively engaged in the broader world (e.g. volunteering, participating in the arts, serving a religious community, etc), youth in this study got the opportunity to develop or cultivate special skills, and they recognized that through these special skills they were able to do something useful for the world around them. For these youth, the opportunity to contribute became personally meaningful, and finding a way of applying special skills to solve personally meaningful social problems is the root of purpose (Damon 2008). As a result of these experiences, the youth began to view themselves through this lens of purpose, and in this way, developing a purpose in life spurred the growth of identity.

However the relationship appears to work in both directions. A second model explains how identity formation can support the ongoing development of purpose (Bronk 2011). As Erikson (1968) predicted, emerging research finds that growth around identity fosters the ongoing development of purpose as individuals' continued engagement leads them to infer an even deeper connection to their purposeful pursuits (Bronk 2011). As young people become more involved in their purposeful work, they can begin to identify themselves by these efforts (e.g. a young environmentalist refers to herself as a "tree hugger;" a deeply religious young woman identifies herself foremost as a "Christian"). In other words, young people's far horizon aims provide them with important information about the content of their emerging identities. Taken together, evidence exists for the mutually reinforcing relationship between purpose and identity development.

The identity capital model (Côté 1996, 1997) similarly proposes that growth in purpose and identity reinforce one another, but it offers a slightly different mechanism for how this relationship functions. The identity capital model, as the name implies, suggests that identity capital can result from purposeful engagement and that it can support the subsequent development of a healthy sense of identity. The identity capital model was introduced to explain the process of identity formation in late-modern, postindustrial societies (Côté 2002), and it suggests that individuals with a clear sense of who they are and of what they hope to accomplish in life are better able to understand and make sense of the world around them. This model includes both predictors and indices of identity consolidation and draws on Erikson's belief that a coherent sense of identity is best facilitated by an agentic orientation in which the person engages in purposeful interaction with the social environment. Discovering purpose appears to help individuals resolve identity "crises" by offering them a meaningful aim toward which they can direct their time, energy, and effort (Burrow and Hill 2011). As a consequence of being engaged in the broader world in a personally meaningful way, individuals develop capital, or resources, that facilitate further growth. Identity capital includes assets or capabilities, such as initiative and efficacy, which are likely to facilitate both the growth of purpose and identity. In fact, purposeful engagement may engender particularly valuable forms of identity capital because it can connect individuals' experiences to meaningful aspects of their identities and engender a sense of efficacy with regards to goal achievement (Burrow and Hill 2011; Burrow et al. 2010; Côté and Levine 2002). In this way, one of the primary benefits of identifying a purpose during adolescence may be that doing so promotes a positive, efficacious sense of identity that can facilitate the transition to adulthood (Burrow et al. 2010).

External Support for Purpose Development It is clear from this preceding discussion that the development of purpose is associated with healthy identity formation. However, only a small percentage of young people today discover and commit to personally meaningful aspirations (Bronk et al. 2010; Damon 2008; Francis 2000; Moran 2009). Consequently, a growing body of empirical research attempts to identify the factors that influence the development of purpose. In particular, researchers have investigated the way adolescents' social relationships (e.g. family, peers, and mentors) and their developmental contexts (e.g. extracurricular, academic, and religious) can foster purpose.

Social Support The presence of a strong social network is one of the most important predictors of purpose. A longitudinal study of adolescents interested in uncovering the antecedents of generativity, a concept that shares with purpose a personally meaningful commitment to issues beyond-the-self, followed a sample of young people from 17- to 23-years of age (Lawford et al. 2005). Results suggest that generative youth are likely to have authoritative parents and to be prosocially engaged in their communities. Underscoring the important role of parents, another study determined that adolescents who go on to develop meaningful purposes are likely to have strong father figures in their lives (Padleford 1974).

Other research suggests that positive relationships with adults outside the family may further support the development of purpose. For instance, a recent study revealed that youth with purpose reported having close, long-term relationships with mentors who helped them discover and pursue their purposes (Bronk 2012). Another study determined that disabled Korean adolescents identified friends and family members as playing a key role in helping them find meaning in their lives (Kim and Kang 2003). Frankl (1959) adamantly believed that individuals could discover purpose even under extremely difficult circumstances. Consistent with this idea, the sample of disabled individuals noted that the challenge of growing up disabled in a culture where most people look down on them provided a difficult, but not impossible, backdrop against which to discover meaning in their lives (Kim and Kang 2003). Additionally, a study of rural adolescents concluded that youth with purpose reported higher levels of social support from parents, mentors, schools, and communities than rural youth without purpose (Bronk,et al. under review). Taken together, these studies offer growing evidence for the important role of social support in the growth of purpose.

Education In addition to spending time with families, most adolescents and emerging adults also spend a significant amount of time in educational contexts. Accordingly, researchers have investigated ways that academic environments can contribute to purpose development. One such study concluded that adolescents and emerging adults in school report higher levels of meaningful instrumental activity than similarly aged young people who are not in school (Maton 1990). This finding suggests that one way schools can contribute to the growth of purpose is by providing students with meaningful opportunities to be engaged.

However, a review of studies examining academic contexts and purpose reveals that the relationship between education and purpose is not an entirely straightforward one. For example, early research, using the Purpose in Life test (PIL), found that college freshman actually reported more purpose than college seniors, suggesting that more education did not equate to more purpose (Crumbaugh and Maholick 1967). Another team of researchers (Laufer et al. 1981), using the same measure of purpose, came to a similar conclusion; among a small sample of older adults, PIL scores did not vary as a function of educational attainment. However, more recent research using Ryff's Psychological Scales of Well-being Purpose sub-scale (Ryff 1989; Ryff and Keyes 1995), has found that as educational attainment increased, purpose scores also increased. Individuals with a college degree scored higher on purpose than individuals with some college who in turn scored higher than individuals with only a high school degree who in turn scored higher than individuals with less than a high school diploma or GED (Ryff and Singer 2008).

The apparent discrepancy may be explained by considering both the nature of the study samples and the timing of each study. Crumbaugh and Maholick (1967) compared college freshman to college seniors. The difference in their level of educational achievement was relatively narrow and could have obscured the results. Further, in the 1960s and 1970s, when the two PIL studies were conducted, a college degree meant something different than it does today. Then most individuals who had completed some college likely would have felt confident that they could pursue their long-term aims and purposes. Today this may not be the case. With the number of manufacturing jobs declining and outsourcing to oversees labor markets increasing, more specialized education is often required not only to earn a living but also to pursue a purpose. The pursuit of service-oriented, career-oriented, and familial purposes is likely to require more education today than it did sixty years ago. If we assume that the more recent finding is more accurate in Western cultures in the twenty-first century, then this is significant. It means that the pursuit of purpose may not be equally available to all people. Opportunities for self-realization may not be evenly distributed throughout society, but instead may only be available via the allocation of educational resources, which enable only some to pursue their aspirations (Dowd 1990; Ryff and Singer 2008). While there are sure to be some exceptions, it seems likely that educational attainment could serve as a gatekeeper of sorts for the pursuit of at least some forms of purpose.

This assumes that rates of purpose will increase as a result of increases in educational attainment, and while there seems to be some evidence for this relationship, the existing evidence is correlational in nature, not causal. That means that the relationship *could* work in the other direction. It *could* be the case that increases in purpose lead to increases in academic achievement. In other words, once individuals know what they want to accomplish they may feel more motivated to work hard in school. Emerging research with adolescents offers some support for this possibility. As discussed in greater depth in Chap. 3 (The Role of Purpose in Optimal Human Development), increases in rates of purpose and internal locus of control have been found to precede increases in grade point averages among students from low-income socioeconomic backgrounds (Pizzolato et al. 2011). Further, students who can articulate their inspiring interests or "sparks," which are potential indicators of purpose, and who find support for pursuing these interests likewise report increased levels of academic achievement (Benson 2008). Additional research is needed to further clarify the directional nature of the relationship between purpose and academic achievement among adolescents, but in short, there is strong evidence that the two are related.

There are a variety of reasons for purpose and academic achievement to be related. One reason likely has to do with future orientation. Young people who have a clear goal toward which they aspire and who are able to make connections between that goal and their education, are more likely to be motivated in the classroom (Damon 2008). A small, but growing body of empirical work supports this claim. First, research finds that young people who have developed or who are in the process of developing a sense of identity tend to hold better-defined educational purposes and have clearer plans for achieving those aims (Berzonsky and Kuk 2000). Educational purpose, or a well-defined and realistic career goal, is associated with career exploration and planning, effective study habits, and self-assuredness. Second, individuals who aspire to professional goals because of what they can do for others or for causes beyond themselves are more likely to report that their schoolwork is personally meaningful (Yeagar and Bundick 2009). Accordingly, we can conclude that youth inspired by purpose are likely to be more motivated and more committed students than youth who lack purpose.

However, while youth with purpose may be more motivated in the classroom, they are not necessarily more intelligent. A study of high ability early and late adolescents concluded that gifted youth commit to life purposes at roughly the same rate and time as more typical youth (Bronk et al. 2010).

Extracurricular and Faith-related Activities Beyond the classroom, researchers have also investigated the role extracurricular and faith-based activities play in the development of purpose. Involvement in community service, arts, or religious activities, appears to be significantly positively associated with the development and maintenance of purpose (Bronk 2012; Maton 1990). Adolescents who pray regularly, whether they go to church or not, are also more likely than adolescents who do not pray to report having a purpose in their lives (Francis and Evans 1996). These findings are highly intuitive. Not only are community service, arts, and religious contexts likely to attract individuals who find purpose in these areas, but these contexts also offer important avenues for purpose development.

It is impossible to discern from existing research if involvement in extracurricular and faith-based activities leads to the development of purpose, or if young people with purposeful interests are drawn to these activities, or if there is a third factor, perhaps friendships or mentoring relationships, that both lead adolescents to these activities and contribute to the growth of purpose. However, it seems likely that involvement in these potentially purposeful activities contributes, at least to some degree, to the development of purpose as these youth are given the opportunity to learn about issues that may interest or concern them. By being engaged in these activities they are afforded the opportunity to discover ways in which their talents make them particularly well suited to acting in potentially meaningful capacities (Bronk 2012; Damon 2008).

Substance abuse Involvement in certain relationships and activities is positively associated with the presence of purpose during adolescence and emerging adulthood, and involvement in other activities is negatively associated with the presence of purpose. For example, adolescents who use drugs or alcohol are less likely to report having a sense of purpose in their lives (Coleman et al. 1986; Minehan et al. 2000; Padleford 1974). Similarly, meaninglessness has been found to mediate the relationship between uncontrollable stress and substance use among adolescents (Newcomb and Harlow 1986) and between depression and self-derogation (Harlow et al. 1986). Clearly drug use is a sign that youth are not on the path to developing a meaningful purpose in life.

Emotions In addition to focusing on potential contributors to the development of purpose during adolescence and emerging adulthood, research has also sought to understand and describe the experience of youth purpose. For instance, certain emotions during adolescence and emerging adulthood are significantly related to the presence of purpose. In particular, youth with purpose tend to report higher levels of, hope and life satifaction (Bronk et al. 2009; Burrow and Hill 2011) than youth without purpose. Along these same lines, youth without purpose are more likely to experience depression (Bigler et al. 2001), anxiety (Ho et al. 2010), and boredom (Fahlman et al. 2009; Drob and Bernard 1988; Bargdill 2000) than youth with purpose. A fuller discussion of the relationship between purpose and indicators of well-being is included in the preceding chapter (Chap. 3, The Role of Purpose in Optimal Human Functioning).

Conceptions of Purpose Given that purpose is associated with healthy developmental outcomes, it is important to know how adolescents and emerging adults conceive of the construct. Asked to define purpose, a sample of college students in the United States said that purpose provides a strong foundation and a clear direction for growth (Hill et al. 2010). Most also noted that it leads to happiness. We can conclude from this that young peoples' conceptions largely align with researchers' conceptions; however, it is interesting to note that youth do not highlight the importance of working toward beyond-the-self aims, as researchers do. Interestingly, a similar study conducted with adults concluded that older participants do conceive of purpose, or at least of meaning, as including this beyond-the-self facet (Wong and Fry 1998). Together these studies point to a possible developmental shift in conceptions of personally meaningful aspirations.

Not only do adolescents conceive of purpose differently than adults, but they also tend to discuss it in different terms. Inhelder and Piaget (1958) found, for example, that in diary musings, youth reflected on other-oriented life aims in ways that were particularly grandiose and lofty. They discussed ways of becoming great thinkers, world leaders, and solution seekers to humanity's deepest philosophical and societal problems. In spite of this- or perhaps because of this- Inhelder and Piaget (1958) concluded that an adolescent's life project may have a "real influence on the individual's later growth, and it may even be that a person discovers in his adolescent jottings an outline of some ideas which he has really fulfilled since" (pp. 334–335). In other words, the commitments made during adolescence and emerging adulthood may shape future aspirations and goals in significant ways.

Theoretical and empirical research on purpose during the adolescent and emerging adult life stages has important implications for how to effectively foster purpose. Many of the same relationships, opportunities, and experiences that support positive youth development in general also appear to support the development of purpose in particular. Accordingly, young people with strong social support, including familial, mentor, and peer relationships, and youth who grow up in supportive developmental contexts, including educational, extracurricular, and religious environments, are both likely to thrive (Benson 2006) and poised to discover purpose (Bronk et al. under review; Bronk 2012).

Midlife

Some adolescents and emerging adults commit to personally meaningful aspirations that are likely to guide their transition into midlife. Purpose can serve as an important source of direction for youth and adults alike. However, rates of purpose tend to drop slightly from their peak in emerging adulthood (Ryff and Singer 2008; Ryff et al. 2004). It is not immediately clear why this drop occurs, but a meta-analysis of 70 studies of purpose suggests that midlife adults may experience age-associated losses in purpose (Pinquart 2002). Some midlife adults may achieve goals that previously gave their lives meaning and wonder what is next. Others may become convinced that certain meaningful aims no longer seem realistically attainable. Still others may find that roles where they had once derived meaning change. Roles, including parenting, caregiving, working, and volunteering, provide important sources of purpose, and if and when these roles disappear, purpose presumably fades.

The drop in rates of purpose during midlife is troubling given that pursuing purpose can offer midlife adults an important route to generativity. Generativity versus stagnation represents Erikson's (1968) seventh stage of psychosocial development, and finding a means of being generative represents the primary developmental task of middle adulthood. During this stage, contributing to society and doing things that benefit future generations becomes increasingly important to adult well-being. Midlife adults who are generative discover meaningful ways of leaving behind a positive legacy. They may do this through parenting, caring for others, or volunteering. These activities are not necessarily generative, but when they are approached with a desire to help future generations, they can generative.

When adults fail to find ways of leaving behind a positive legacy, they are likely to stagnate, and stagnant individuals tend to experience a sense of disconnect from their communities and societies.

Parenting and grandparenting represent common sources of purpose in midlife (Hughes 2006). In most societies, people associate parenting with happiness and well-being, but research, elaborated upon more fully in the preceding chapter, finds that midlife parents actually report feeling less happy than non-parents; however, they tend to report that their lives are more meaningful than similarly aged adults who do not have children (Umberson and Gove 1989). Well versed in the daily challenges involved in child rearing, midlife adults may not always enjoy the task, but they generally value the purpose derived from the role (Hughes 2006).

However, parenting, like other potential sources of purpose, is not necessarily meaningful. To a large degree, whether parenting is experienced as purposeful depends on how well parents feel they have fulfilled the role. Parents who believe they have parented successfully, and that their adult children have "turned out" well academically and professionally, are significantly more likely to report that being a parent imbues their lives with purpose than parents who do not feel their adult children have succeeded in these socially valued realms (Ryff et al. 1994, p. 195).

Perhaps because of the potential source of purpose provided by the parenting role, research finds that a loss in reproductive ability can trigger a drop in purpose. Most women identify themselves, at least in part, by their role as mothers, but during midlife women go through menopause, and researchers have found that premenopausal women report higher purpose scores than perimenopausal women who in turn report higher purpose scores than postmenopausal women (Deeks and McCabe 2004). One explanation for this trend may have to do with the women's perceived change in their social roles. Consistent with this hypothesis, premenopausal women report feeling most positive about their social roles, and postmenopausal women are more likely than both perimenopausal and premenopausal women to report that they do not fill any significant social roles. These findings underscore the importance of social roles as potential sources of midlife purpose.

Another role that many midlife adults assume is that of caregiver, watching over friends, relatives, and aging parents. Similar to the research on parenting, research also finds that caregivers often report feeling higher distress and a greater sense of burden than non-caregivers, but despite this, caregivers typically report higher rates of purpose than non-caregivers (Marks et al. 2002). In combination with the parenting results (Umberson and Gove 1989), this study suggests that the midlife experience of purpose, while meaningful, may not always be pleasant.

In addition to finding purpose through parenting and caregiving, midlife adults also report finding purpose in other social roles. For example, adult participants were asked to write about, rank, and give an example of the three most significant sources of meaning in their lives. Though most adults reported finding meaning in their relationships, presumably including relationships with children and those for whom they care, they also reported finding meaning in their roles as workers and volunteers (DeVogler and Ebersole 1981).

From this review, we can conclude that social roles provide an important avenue for purpose in midlife. It is also evident that purpose in midlife serves an important generative function that is not as salient at other stages in the lifespan. Lastly, it is clear that while purpose tends to be associated with happiness in earlier stages, this is not always the case in midlife.

Late Adulthood

Research on purpose in later adulthood focuses primarily on the construct's role in supporting positive health. Committed to the idea that positive health is "more than the absence of illness" (World Health Organization as cited in Ryff and Singer 2008), Carol Ryff and Burton Singer have investigated the role of purpose in promoting physical and psychological well-being in later adulthood. Ryff and Singer (2008) find that three principles underlie the formulation of positive mental health. First, they argue that positive health is not so much a medical as a philosophical state that requires a deep articulation of the meaning of a good life. Second, human wellness is at once about the mind, body, and interconnections between the two. Third, positive human health is ultimately about being fully engaged in the process of living.

Well-being in later adulthood, Ryff and Singer argue, is manifest in eudaimonia, which represents Aristotle's conception of the greatest good: the full realization of personal potential (Ryff and Singer 2008; Ryff et al. 2004). Aristotelian the concept of eudaimonia is discussed in preceding chapters, but in short Ryff's theory of well-being suggests that along with environmental mastery, positive relationships, personal growth, autonomy, and self-acceptance, having a purpose in life is a critical component of eudaimonia. While each of these six factors contributes to well-being, a variety of empirical studies suggest that having a purpose in life is a particularly important facet of eudamonia (Ryff and Singer 2008).

Not only is purpose a key component of older adults' psychological well-being, but it also appears to play an important role in their physical health. As discussed in greater detail in Chap. 3 (The Role of Purpose in Optimal Human Functioning), an emerging body of research using a variety of measures of purpose concludes that purpose and purposeful engagement are modestly but consistently associated with improved markers of physical health (Kass et al. 1991; Petrie and Azariah 1990; Reker et al. 1987; Ryff et al. 2004) and longevity for older adults (Boyle et al. 2009).

However, despite the positive role of purpose in later adulthood, the construct is even less prevalent than in preceding stages. From emerging adulthood to midlife the decrease in the prevalence of purpose is slight, but from midlife to later adulthood the drop is more significant (Pinquart 2002; Ryff 1995; Ryff and Singer 2008; Ryff et al. 2004). Rates of purpose among individuals 85 years of age and older is particularly low (Hedberg et al. 2010), and given that purpose plays a key role in well-being, this finding is disturbing (Ryff and Singer 2008). The drop has been blamed on decreasing opportunities for purposeful engagement. Older adults need the autonomy to choose and pursue projects that are personally meaningful, but many of these opportunities evaporate in later adulthood.

During midlife, individuals often find purpose in their social roles as parents, caregivers, workers, and volunteers. However, if some of these roles begin to fade in midlife, they often begin to disappear completely in later adulthood. Adult children move out, retirement replaces work, and health concerns may limit caregiving and volunteer efforts. Potentially purposeful roles for older adults are largely lacking in today's society. Sociologists have termed this "the structural lag problem" (Riley et al. 1994), and it describes the current situation in which contemporary social institutions lag behind the added years of life that many now experience (Ryff and Singer 2008).

While the decline in rates of purpose from midlife to later adulthood is problematic, it is still relatively modest, and some older adults do manage to maintain purpose in this stage of life. A meta-analysis of studies of purpose revealed that older adults who report higher levels of purpose tend to be more socially integrated and have stronger, more positive relationships than older adults who lack purpose (Pinquart 2002). Older adults who live in private homes and apartments report higher levels of purpose than those who live in nursing homes or institutional settings (Laufer et al. 1981). Purposeful older adults are also more likely to be employed, to have better health, to have a higher level of educational attainment, and to be married (Pinquart 2002). Interestingly, among older adults consistent contact with family is a stronger predictor of purpose than consistent contact with friends.

In addition to finding purpose in their families, older adults also report finding purpose in volunteer work. Volunteer opportunities for older adults used to be extremely rare, but today they are becoming more common as society slowly begins to recognize older adults as resources to be cultivated. SeniorCorps, for example, is similar to AmeriCorps but geared for older adults. The organization connects hundreds of thousands of older adults with service opportunities across the United States. This is promising, as older adults who engage in formal volunteering report higher levels of life purpose than those who do not (Greenfield and Marks 2004).

Helping older adults pursue their purposes in life is an important, but underappreciated aim, especially in healthcare contexts. In working with older adults, health care workers often focus on activities of daily living and largely neglect activities of meaningful living. In so doing, they are ignoring purpose, which may be a protective health factor in this later adult life stage (Ryff and Singer 1998). Individuals with positive purposes tend to take better care of themselves; "simply put, taking good care of oneself in terms of daily health practices presupposes a life that is worth taking care of" (Ryff and Singer 1998, p. 22).

In sum, purpose in later adulthood is rare, but still vitally important to psychological and physical health and longevity. However, the availability of potentially purposeful social roles and the ability to fill these roles represent important pre-requisites to pursing purpose late in life.

Purpose Across the Lifespan

As a developmental construct, purpose supports healthy human functioning across much of the lifespan. It can serve as an important source of guidance and direction, influencing the way adolescents, emerging adults, midlife adults, and later adults allocate their time, energy, and other psychological resources. Interestingly, sources of purpose remain largely stable across the lifespan. (Prager 1996). For a fuller discussion of the origins and sources of purpose, please refer to Chap. 5 (Origins of and Supports for Purpose).

However, while the overarching function of purpose is consistent across the lifespan, the way individuals pursue and discuss their life purposes changes over time (Bronk 2012). In childhood, purpose is characterized by purposeful engagement rather than by purposeful commitments, as children are likely to be engaged in a variety of activities that may eventually turn into purposes. If children begin to conceive of a purpose at all, it is likely to be in a decidedly concrete, focused, and present-oriented manner (VanDyke and Elias 2007). Intentional purposeful commitments begin to take form in adolescence and emerging adulthood, when young people being to reflect on who they hope to become and what they hope to accomplish in their lives. Toward the end of emerging adulthood, when most young people have resolved issues of identity, rates of purpose peak (Bronk et al. 2010; Damon 2008; Meier and Edwards 1974; Ryff 1995; Ryff et al. 2003).

From their high point in emerging adulthood, rates of purpose drop slightly into midlife and more significantly into later adulthood, as opportunities to be purposefully engaged diminish (Ryff 1995; Ryff et al. 2003). However, midlife adults who maintain purpose are likely to find it a personally meaningful avenue for generative activity. Pursing purpose in midlife can provide adults with a way to be productive, creative, and to leave behind a positive legacy. Midlife adults often find purpose in their social roles as parents, workers, caregivers, and volunteers. For later adults, having a purpose may serve as a protective factor buffering them from psychological and physical health problems (Ryff and Singer 2008).

Not only does the prevalence of purpose change throughout the lifespan, but so too does the experience of searching for purpose. As discussed in the preceding chapter, the search for purpose is associated with life satisfaction during adolescence and emerging adulthood, but not during midlife, when adults are expected to have completed this search (Bronk et al. 2009).

Regardless of when individuals discover purpose, it is likely that certain triggering incidents or significant life events will be associated with the experience (Baum and Stewart 1990; Bronk 2012). Adolescents and emerging adults point to triggering events in the media, discovering new opportunities to serve others in meaningful ways, and changes in life circumstances as significant moments in the development of purpose (Bronk 2012). Similarly, midlife adults often cite major life changes, such as getting married, becoming parents, having accidents, experiencing illness, losing loved ones, finding new jobs, or getting divorced, as events that prompt the development of purpose (Baum and Stewart 1990). Interestingly, even negative life events, as Frankl (1959) predicted, appear to inspire positive purposes.

Similar to triggering events, life transitions can also contribute to the growth and evolution of purposes. A longitudinal study of youth determined that purposes often expanded and shifted as a result of natural transitions in the lifespan (Bronk 2012). For example, in some cases transitions to college or work exposed youth in the sample to new resources and mentors who redirected their approach to pursuing their personally meaningful aims. In other cases, new environments and new people challenged the young people's ways of thinking about their purposes. Over the course of the five-year study, however, while many of the youth reported changes in the way they pursued their purpose, none reported changing the nature of their personally meaningful aspirations.

Purpose as a State and Trait Underlying this discussion of purpose across the lifespan is the assumption that a purpose represents an enduring aspect of who one is. The bulk of the research on purpose points to the construct's stability over time. For example, a series of studies using different measures of purpose have found that life meaning is stable over two-weeks (Meaning in Life questionnaire; Steger et al. 2006), two months (Meaning in Life questionnaire; Steger et al. 2008), one-year (Meaning in Life questionnaire; Steger and Kashdan 2007), and two-years (Sense of Coherence scale; Antonovsky 1987). Findings that suggest purpose represents an enduring aspect of identity (Bronk 2011; Damon 2008) further highlight the trait-like characteristic of the construct. However, a handful of studies have also concluded that levels of purposeful commitment can, to some degree anyway, wax and wane in response to contextual factors and life events. For instance, the depth of commitment to purpose has been found to peak within a week of religious conversion and to drop in the weeks that follow (Paloutzian 1981). Similarly, rates of purpose appear to dip following experiences of social exclusion (Stillman et al. 2009) and to increase following life transitions (Ryff and Singer 1998). These findings point to the state-like characteristics of purpose.

While the bulk of the evidence supports the enduring nature of purpose, it is clear that this characteristic is influenced to some degree anyway by life events and circumstances. It seems plausible that the depth of commitment may influence the degree to which this characteristic is stable over time, A more central purpose may be more stable. Empirical work is needed to test this possibility.

While it is evident that purpose grows and changes across the lifespan, it is not entirely clear how its development—or the likelihood that it will develop at all– is influenced by contextual and environmental factors. The following chapter synthesizes existing theoretical and empirical research on opportunities, experiences, and social and ecological supports for the development of purpose over time.

References

Antonovsky, A. (1987). *Unraveling the mystery of health.* San Francisco: Jossey Bass.

Arnett, J. J. (2000). Emerging adulthood: A theory of development from the late teens through the twenties. *American Psychologists, 55,* 469–480.

Bargdill, R. W. (2000). The study of boredom. *Journal of Phenomenological Psychology, 31,* 188–219.

Baum, S. K., & Stewart, R. B. (1990). Sources of meaning through the lifespan. *Psychological Reports, 67,* 3–14.

Benson, P. L. (2006). *All kids are our kids: What communities must do to raise caring and responsible children and adolescents, 2nd Edition.* San Francisco: Jossey Bass.

Benson, P. L. (2008). *Sparks: How parents can help ignite the hidden strengths of teenagers.* San Francisco: Jossey Bass.

Berzonsky, M. D., & Kuk, L. S. (2000). Identity status, identity processing style, and the transition to university. *Journal of Adolescent Research, 15,* 81–98.

Bigler, M., Neimeyer, G. J., & Brown, E. (2001). The divided self revisited: Effects of self-concept clarity and self-concept differentiation on psychological adjustment. *Journal of Social & Clinical Psychology, 20,* 396–415.

Boyle, P. A., Barnes, L. L., Buchman, A. S., & Bennett, D. A. (2009). Purpose in life is associated with mortality among community-dwelling older persons. *Psychosomatic Medicine, 71,* 574–579.

Bronk, K. C. (2011). Portraits of purpose: The role of purpose in identity formation. A special issue on instructing for and supporting youth purpose in. *New Directions in Youth Development, 132,* 31–44.

Bronk, K. C. (2012). A grounded theory of youth purpose. *Journal of Adolescent Research,* 27, 78–109. http://dx.doi.org/10.1177/0743558411412958.

Burrow, A., & Hill, P. L. (2011). Purpose as a form of identity capital for positive youth adjustment. *Developmental Psychology, 47*(4), 1196–1206.

Bronk, K. C., Hill, P., Lapsley, D., K., Talib, T., & Finch, W. H. (2009). Purpose, hope, and life satisfaction in three age groups. *Journal of Positive Psychology, 4*(6), 500–510.

Bronk, K. C., Finch, W. H., & Talib, T. (2010). Purpose among high ability adolescents. *High Ability Studies, 21*(2), 133–145.

Bronk, K. C., Finch, H. W., Kollman, J. & Youngs, A., (under review, Oct. 2012). Ecological and social support for rural youth purpose. Submitted to *Journal of Happiness Studies.*

Burrow, A. L., O'Dell, A. C., & Hill, P. L. (2010). Profiles of a developmental asset: Youth purpose as a context for hope and well-being. *Journal of Youth and Adolescence, 39,* 1265–1273.

Coleman, S., Kaplan, J., & Downing, R. (1986). Life cycle and loss: The spiritual vacuum of heroin addiction. *Family Process, 25,* 5–23.

Côté, J. E. (1996). Sociological perspectives on identity formation: The culture-identity link and identity capital. *Journal of Adolescence, 19,* 417–428.

Côté, J. E. (1997). An empirical test of the identity capital model. *Journal of Adolescence, 20,* 577–597.

Côté, J. E. (2000). *Arrested adulthood: The changing nature of identity and maturity in the late-modern world.* New York: New York University Press.

Côté, J. E. (2002). The role of identity capital in the transition to adulthood: The individualization thesis examined. *Journal of Youth Studies, 5*(2), 117–134.

Côté, J. E., & Allahar, A. (1996). *Generation on hold: Coming of age in the late twentieth century.* New York: New York University Press.

Côté, J. E., & Levine, C. (1982). Marcia and Erikson: The relationship among ego identity statuses, neuroticism, dogmatism, and purpose in life. *Journal of Youth and Adolescence, 12*(1), 43–53.

Côté, J. E., & Levine, C. (2002). *Identity formation, agency, and culture: A social psychological synthesis.* Mahwah, NJ: Lawrence Erlbaum.

Crumbaugh, J. C., & Maholick, L. T. (1967). An experimental study in existentialism: The psychometric approach to Frankl's concept of noogenic neurosis. In V. E. Frankl (Ed.), *Psychotherapy and existentialism* (pp. 183–197). New York: Washington Square Press.

Damon, W. (2008). *The path to purpose: Helping our children find their calling in life*. New York: Free Press.

Deeks, A. A., & McCabe, M. P. (2004). Well-being and menopause: An investigation of purpose in life, self-acceptance, and social role in premenopausal, perimenopausal, and post menopausal women. *Quality of Life Research, 13,* 389–398.

DeVogler, K. L., & Ebersole, P. (1981). Adults' meaning in life. *Psychological Reports, 49,* 87–90.

Dowd, J. J. (1990). Ever since Durkheim: The socialization of human development. *Human Development, 33,* 138–159.

Drob, S. L., & Bernard, H. S. (1988). The bored patient: A developmental existential perspective. *Psychotherapy Patient, 3*(3-4), 63–73.

Erikson, E. H. (1968). *Identity: youth and crisis*. New York: W. W. Norton.

Erikson, E. H. (1980). *Identity and the life cycle (paperback)*. New York: W.W. Norton & Company Inc.

Fahlman, S. A., Mercer, K. B., Gaskovski, P., Eastwood, A. E., & Eastwood, J. D. (2009) Does a lack of life meaning cause boredom? Results from psychometric, longitudinal, and experimental analyses. *Journal of Social and Clinical Psychology, 28*(3), 307–340.

Fegg, M., Kramer, M., Bausewin, C., & Borasio, F. D. (2007). Meaning in life lin the Federal Republic of Germany: Results of a representative survey with the SCHEDULE for Meaning in Life Evaluation (SMiLE). *Health and Quarterly of Life Outcomes, 5,* 59–66.

Francis, L. J. (2000). The relationship between bible reading and purpose in life among 13-15-year olds. *Mental Health, Religion, and Culture*, *3*(1), 27–36.

Francis, L. J., & Evans, T. E. (1996). The relationship between personal prayer and purpose in life among churchgoing and non-churchgoing twelve-to-fifteen-year-olds in the UK. *Religious Education, 91*(1), 9–21.

Frankl, V. E. (1959). *Man's search for meaning: An introduction to logotherapy*. Boston: Beacon.

French, S., & Joseph, S. (1999). Religiosity and its association with happiness, purpose in life, and self-actualization. *Mental Health, Religion, & Culture, 2,* 117–120.

Fry, P. S. (1998). The development of personal meaning and wisdom in adolescence: A reexamination of moderating and consolidating factors an influences. In P. T. P. Wong (Ed.), *The human quest for meaning: A handbook of psychological research and clinical application* (2nd edition). (pp. 91–110). New York: Routledge.

Gillham, J., Adams-Deutsch, Z., Werner, J., Reivich, K., Coulter-Heindl, V., Linkins, M., Winder, B., Peterson, C., Park, N., Abenavoli, R., Contero, A., & Seligman, M. E. P. (2011). Character strengths predict subjective well-being during adolescence. *Journal of Positive Psychology, 6*(1), 31–44. doi: 10.1080/17439760.2010.536773.

Greenfield, E. A., & Marks, N. F. (2004). Formal volunteering as a protective factor for older adults' psychological well-being. *The Journal of Gerontology Series B: Psychological Sciences and Social Sciences, 59B*(5), 258–264.

Harlow, L. L., Newcomb, M. D., & Bentler, P. M. (1986). Depression, self-derogation, substance use, and suicide ideation: Lack of purpose in life as a meditational factor. *Journal of Clinical Psychology, 42*(1), 5–21.

Hedberg, P., Gudtafson, Y., & Brulin, C. (2010). Purpose in life among men and women aged 85 years and older. *The International Journal of Aging and Human Development, 70*(3), 213–229.

Hill, P. L., & Burrow, A. (2012). Viewing purpose through an Eriksonian lens. *Identity: An International Journal of Theory and Research, 12*(2), 74–91.

Hill, P. L., Burrow, A., O'Dell, A. C., & Thornton, M. A. (2010). Classifying adolescents' conceptions of purpose in life. *Journal of Positive Psychology, 5*(6), 466–473.

Ho, M. Y., Cheung, F. M., & Cheung, S. F. (2010). The role of meaning in life and optimism in promoting well-being. *Personality and individual differences, 48*(5), 658–663.

Hughes, M. (2006). Affect, meaning, and quality of life. *Social Forces, 85*(2), 611–629.

Inhelder, B., & Piaget, J. (1958). *The growth of logical thinking from childhood to adolescence*. New York: Basic Books.
Ishida, R., & Okada, M. (2006). Effects of a firm purpose in life on anxiety and sympathetic nervous activity caused by emotional stress: Assessment by psychological method. *Stress and health: Journal of the International Society for the Investigation of Stress, 22*(4), 275–281.
Kass, J. D., Friedman, R., Leserman, J., Caudill, M., Zuttermeister, P. C., & Benson, H. (1991). An inventory of positive psychological attitudes with potential relevance to health outcomes: Validation and preliminary testing. *Behavioral Medicine, 17*(3), 121–129.
Kim, S. J., & Kang, K. A. (2003). Meaning of life for adolescents with a physical disability in Korea. *Journal of Advanced Nursing, 43*(2), 145–155.
Lawford, H., Pratt, M. W., Hunsberger, B., & Pancer, S. M. (2005). Adolescent Generativity: A Longitudinal Study of Two Possible Contexts for Learning Concern for Future Generations. *Journal of Research on Adolescence, 15*(3), 261–273.
Laufer, W. S., Laufer, E. A., & Laufer, L. S. (1981). Purpose in life and occupational interest in a gerontological sheltered workshop. *Journal of Clinical Psychology, 37*(4), 424–426.
Lewis, C. A., Lanigan, C., Joseph, S., & de Fockert, J. (1997). Religiosity and happiness: No evidence for an association among undergraduates. *Personality and Individual Differences, 22,* 119–121.
Marcia, J. E. (1966). Development and validation of ego-identity status. *Journal of Personality and Social Psychology, 3,* 551–558.
Mariano, J. M., & Vaillant, G. E. (2012). Purpose among the "Greatest Generation." *Journal of Positive Psychology*. DOI:10.1080/17439760.2012.686624.
Marks, N. F., Lambert, J. D., & Choi, H. (2002). Transitions to caregiving, gender, and psychological well-being: A perspective U.S. national study. *Journal of Marriage and Family, 64,* 657–67.
Markstrom, C. A., Berman, R. C., Sabino, V. M., & Turner, B. (1998). The ego virtue of fidelity as a psocohosocial rite of passage in the transition from adolescence to adulthood. *Child & Youth Care Forum, 27*(5), 337–354.
Martinez, R. O., & Dukes, R. L. (1997). The effects of ethnic identity, ethnicity, and gender on adolescent well-being. *Journal of Youth and Adolescence, 26*(5), 503–516.
Maton, K. K. (1990). Meaningful involvement in instrumental activity and well-being: Studies of older adolescents and at risk urban teen-agers. *American Journal of Community Psychology, 18*(2), 297–320.
McLean, K. C., & Pratt, M. W. (2006). Life's little (and big) lessons: Identity statuses and meaning-making in the turning point narratives of emerging adults. *Developmental Psychology, 42*(4), 714–722.
Meier, A., & Edwards, H. (1974). Purpose-in-life Test: Age and sex differences. *Journal of Clinical Psychology, 30,* 384–386.
Minehan, J., Newcomb, M., & Galaif, E. (2000). Predictors of adolescent drug use: Cognitive abilities, coping strategies, and purpose in life. *Journal of Child and Adolescent Substance Abuse, 10,* 33–52.
Moran, S. (2009). Purpose: Giftedness in intrapersonal intelligence. *High Ability Studies, 20*(2), 143–159. DOI:10.1080/13598130903358501.
Newcomb, M. D., & Harlow, L. L. (1986). Life events and substance use among adolescents: Mediating effects of perceived loss of control and meaninglessness in life. *Journal of Personality and Social Psychology, 51*(3), 564–577.
Padelford, B. L. (1974). The relationship between drug involvement and purpose in life. *Journal of Clinical Psychology, 30*(3), 303–305.
Paloutzian, R. F. (1981). Purpose in life and value changes following conversion. *Journal of Personality and Social Psychology, 41*(6), 1153–1160.
Peterson, C., Parks, N. S., & Seligman, M. E. P. (2005). Orientations to happiness and life satisfaction: The full life versus the empty life. *Journal of Happiness Studies, 6,* 25–41.
Petrie, K., & Azariah, R. (1990). Health-promoting variables as predictors of response to a brief pain management program. *Clinical Journal of Pain, 6*(1), 43–46.

Pinquart, M. (2002). Creating and maintaining purpose in life in old age: A meta-analysis. *Ageing international, 27*(2), 90–114.
Pizzolato, J. E., Brown, E. L., & Kanny, M. A. (2011). Purpose plus: Supporting youth purpose, control, and academic achievement. *New Directions for Youth Development, 132,* 75–88.
Prager, E. (1996). Exploring personal meaning in an age-differentiated Australian sample: Another look at the Sources of Meaning Profile (SOMP). *Journal of Aging Studies, 10*(2), 117–136.
Reker, G. T., Peacock, E. J., & Wong, P. T. P. (1987). Meaning and purpose in life and well-being: A life-span perspective. *Journal of Gerontology, 42*(1), 44–49.
Riley, M. W., Kahn, R. L., & Foner, A. (1994). *Age and structural lag: Society's failure to provide meaningful opportunities in work, family, and leisure*. New York: Wiley.
Ryff, C. D. (1989). Scales of psychological well-being. University of Wisconsin Institute on Aging. *Journal of Personality and Social Psychology, 57,* 1069–1081.
Ryff, C. D. (1995). Psychological well-being in adult life. *Current Directions in Psychological Science, 4,* 99–104.
Ryff, C. D., & Keyes, C. L. (1995). The structure of psychological well-being revisited. *Journal of Personality and Social Psychology, 69*(4), 719–27.
Ryff, C. D., & Singer, B. H. (2008). Know thyself and become what you are: A eudaimonic approach to psychological well-being. *Journal of Happiness Studies, 9,* 13–39.
Ryff, C. D., Lee, Y. H., Essex, M. J., & Schmutte, P. S. (1994). My children and me: Midlife evaluations of grown children and self. *Psychology and Aging, 9*(2), 195–205.
Ryff, C. D., & Singer, B. H. (1998). The role of purpose in life and personal growth in positive human health. In P. T. P. Wong (Ed.), *The human quest for meaning: A handbook of psychological research and applications (2nd ed.)* (pp. 213–235). New York: Routledge.
Ryff, C. D., Keyes, C. L. M., & Hughes, D. L. (2003). Status inequalities, perceived discrimination, and eudaimonic well-being: The challenges of minority life hone purpose and growth? *Journal of Health and Social Behavior, 44,* 275–291.
Ryff, C. D., Singer, B., & Love, G. D. (2004). Positive health: Connecting well-being with biology. Philosophical Transactions Royal Society London B, Biological Sciences, 359, 1383-1394. DOI:10.1098/rstb.2004.1521
Schwartz, S. J. (2007). The structure of identity consolidation: Multiple correlated constructs or one superordinate construct? *Identity: An International Journal of Theory and Research, 7,* 27–49.
Schwartz, S. J., Côté, J. E., & Arnett, J. J. (2005). Identity and agency in emerging adulthood: Two developmental routes in the individuation process. *Youth and Society, 37,* 201–229.
Schwartz, S. J., & Montgomery, M. J. (2002). Similarities or differences in identity development? The impact of acculturation and gender on identity process and outcomes. *Journal of Youth and Adolescence, 31,* 359–372.
Seligman, M. E. P. (2011). *Flourish: A visionary new understanding of happiness and well-being.* New York: Free Press.
Steger, M. F., Frazier, P., Oishi, S., & Kaler, M. (2006). The Meaning in Life Questionnaire: Assessing the presence of and search for meaning in life. *Journal of Counseling Psychology, 53,* 80–93.
Steger, M. F., & Kashdan, T. B. (2007). Stability and specificity of meaning in life and life satisfaction over one year. *Journal of Happiness Studies, 8,* 161–179.
Steger, M. F., Kawabata, Y., Shimai, S., & Otake, K. (2008). The meaningful life in Japan and the United States: Levels and correlates of meaning in life. *Journal of Research in Personality, 42,* 660–678.
Stillman, T. F., Baumeister, R. F., Lambert, N., Crescioni, A. W., DeWall, C. N., & Fincham, F. D. (2009). Alone and without purpose: Life loses meaning following social exclusion. *Journal of Experimental Social Psychology, 45,* 686–94.
Umberson, D., & Gove, W. R. (1989). "Parenthood and Psychological Well-Being: Theory, measurement, and stage in the family life course. *Journal of Family Issues, 10*(4), 440–462.
VanDyke, C. J., & Elias, M. J. (2007). How forgiveness, purpose, and religiosity are related to the mental health and well-being of youth. *Mental Health, Religion, & Culture, 10*(4), 395–415.

Vleioras, G., & Bosma, H. A. (2005). Are identity styles important for psychological well-being? *Journal of Adolescence, 28,* 397–409.

Wong, P. T. P. (1998). Implicit theories of meaningful life and the development of the personal meaning profile. In P. T. P. Wong, & P. S. Fry (Eds.), *The human quest for meaning: A handbook of psychological research and clinical applications* (pp. 111–140). Mahwah: Lawrence Erlbaum Associates.

Wong, P. T. P., & Fry, P. S. (1998). *The human quest for meaning: A handbook of psychological research and clinical applications.* Mahwan: Lawrence Erlbaum Associates.

Yeager, D. M., & Bundick, M. (2009). The role of purposeful work goals in promoting meaning in life and in schoolwork during adolescence. *Journal of Adolescent Research, 24*(4), 423–452.

Zika, S., & Chamberlain, K. (1992). On the relation between meaning in life and psychological well-being. *British Journal of Psychology, 83,* 133–145.

Chapter 5
Origins of and Supports for Purpose

Psychological attention and empirical research on purpose are relatively recent phenomenan. A growing body of theoretical and empirical research has focused on what constitutes purpose, on the close correspondence between purpose and identity development, and on the positive correlates of leading a life of purpose. However, comparatively little research has focused on how purposes are discovered or on how they are pursued over time. Consequently, we know relatively little about how to effectively foster this important construct. Few programs, whether in religious, extracurricular, career, or school-based settings, explicitly and intentionally teach people how to find a purpose for their lives (Koshy and Mariano 2011). However, results from a handful of intervention and longitudinal studies point to likely features of effective programs. Based on these studies, it is clear that ecological and social support is critical to the development of purpose (Bronk 2012; Bronk et al., under review; Dik et al. 2011; Pizzolato et al. 2011). An examination of the small body of empirical studies focused on fostering purpose coupled with theoretical research from related topics, sheds important light on how parents, teachers, and other adults concerned with the well-being of young people can effectively help youth discover meaningful purposes for their lives.

Evolutionary Basis for Purpose

While the bulk of this chapter focuses on how to support the development of purpose, it also aims to understand why individuals are concerned with purpose in the first place. Developing a purpose may seem contradictory to evolutionary and biological views of humanity, but in fact researchers have proposed several explanations for how discovering and pursuing purpose may have been evolutionarily adaptive. Different evolutionary theories highlight different aspects of purpose and link them to our evolutionary past in varied ways. Problem solving, goal directedness, and service to the world beyond-the-self are all aspects of purpose that have been singled out as potentially having evolutionary roots.

K. C. Bronk, *Purpose in Life*, DOI 10.1007/978-94-007-7491-9_5,

A recent theory focuses on the role of purpose in solving evolutionary problems (Boyd 2009). According to this perspective, "evolution creates purpose" (p. 24). Put another way, in the course of generating life, evolution creates problems that must be solved, and in solving these problems, individuals often discover meaningful purposes for their lives. Boyd offers two examples of how this may work in practice.

The first has to do with the nature of intelligence and purpose. Throughout our evolutionary past, humans have become increasingly intelligent, which has allowed us to respond flexibly to circumstances and to solve problems not only according to successful old routines, but also in novel ways. One of the important forms of intelligence we have developed is social intelligence or social cognition. Social cognition allows people to be self-aware and to put themselves in others' positions. This of course confers many advantages as individuals are better able to predict others' behaviors, but it also means people can imagine their own deaths and the world without them. To deal with this potential source of anxiety and distress, people have frequently concluded that they continue in some form after death. Based on this belief, nearly all cultures have created stories about what happens to people once they die, and these stories serve as the basis for religion and corresponding religious purposes. In this way, developing a religious purpose may represent an evolutionarily adaptive response to the problem of impending death.

The second example Boyd offers has to do with creative purposes. Human beings have highly evolved brains, which has allowed us to become super-predators and to dominate our environment. We require relatively little time to obtain food, and therefore we find ourselves with a significant amount of time to spend on other activities. During these times of leisure and security, people often engage in cognitive play, which can take the form of art. Art appeals to our appetite for potentially meaningful patterned information, engages our attention in a self-rewarding way, and encourages us to strengthen the processing power of our minds. Because it appeals to our cognitive preferences, art is inherently rewarding. We have built-in incentives to generate art; its effects are pleasing, and meaningful in themselves. In this way, artistic and other creative purposes represent evolutionarily adaptive responses to the problem of boredom. According to Boyd's (2009) view, purpose has developed as a natural outgrowth of intelligence and creativity, and it is evolutionarily adaptive in that it represents an important means of solving uniquely human problems.

While Boyd's (2009) theory proposes that purpose serves an evolutionarily adaptive problem-solving role, other theorists argue that the goal orientation inherent in purpose may have been particularly adaptive in our evolutionary past. In other words, the search for meaning and purpose may be rooted in biology to the extent that goal striving is a biological imperative of living organisms (Klinger 1998). This theory argues that it is people's cognitive and symbolic capacities that have elevated this biological drive to the transcendent experience of purpose. Similarly, it is our emotional reaction to goal striving that results in the affective richness of purpose. In this way, cognition and emotion are intricately related to life goals and contribute to the experience of purposeful living.

Both of the preceding perspectives focus on the individual as the unit of analysis. Others have argued that to understand the evolutionary basis of purpose, we must consider not the individual but the group as the unit of analysis (Nanay 2010). The latter focus is particularly concerned with purposes that include a desire to act in service to the broader world and on behalf of causes beyond-the-self. The individual organism benefits from natural selection. Accordingly, acts that benefit the self are adaptive, but acts that do not benefit the self, such as altruistic or beyond-the-self acts, can be maladaptive, unless they are reciprocated. The adaptability of altruistic or purposeful behavior only becomes clear when it is considered from the perspective of the group. While purposeful acts that benefit the world beyond-the-self may not benefit the individual, they do benefit the group. Generally, these actions increase group cohesion, and the individual members of cohesive groups are more likely to survive over time. From this group perspective, pursuing a beyond-the-self purpose, whether its aim is improvement of one's family, community, or other social group, may be biologically adaptive.

We can conclude from these theories that in a variety of ways, purpose, or at least key components of the construct, appear to have evolutionary bases. It can be argued that the problem-solving capacity, goal orientation aspect, and beyond-the-self components of purpose all serve important evolutionary functions.

Developmental Origins of Purpose

While an evolutionary perspective on purpose reveals much about *why* individuals may develop aspirations, it does not tell us much about *how* they go about doing so. Fortunately, an emerging body of theoretical and empirical research illuminates the process of discovering and committing to personally meaningful long-term aims. This research highlights the role of experiences, opportunities, and other social and ecological supports in the development of purpose.

Opportunities and experiences in childhood can plant the seeds for the future growth of purpose. As discussed in greater detail in Chap. 4 (Purpose across the Lifespan), children lack the cognitive structures required to search for and commit to purposes (VanDyke and Elias 2007); however, a longitudinal study of purpose exemplars revealed that at least some youth who go on to lead lives of purpose first became active in these areas during middle and late childhood (Bronk 2012). Other retrospective studies of purpose conclude that individuals who report more positive experiences in childhood are more likely to discover purposes later in life (Ishida and Okada 2006; Mariano and Vaillant 2012). These findings suggest that contextual factors associated with childhood can influence the likelihood that an individual will develop a purpose later in life.

What is more, a growing body of empirical studies concludes that contextual variables in adolescence and emerging adulthood can similarly increase the chances that youth will discover purposes for their lives. This is hopeful news, given that despite the positive role of purpose, relatively few young people actually report committing to personally meaningful aims (Bronk et al. 2010; Bronk et al. 2009; Damon 2008; Francis 2000; Moran 2009). It is heartening to find that experiences, opportunities, and certain ecological and social supports can increase the likelihood that an individual will develop a meaningful purpose in life.

Before addressing ways outside forces may influence the growth of purpose, however, it is important to reiterate that purpose ultimately comes from within. No one can foist a purpose on another, and there is no sure fire way of ensuring that a particular individual will develop purpose. Purpose only emerges when an individual discovers and commits to pursuing a personally meaningful aim. Still, empirical studies reveal that allowing youth to participate in certain activities, providing them with appropriate guidance, and encouraging them to engage in reflection can increase the odds that they will discover such an aspiration.

Opportunities and Experiences that Foster Purpose

One key step to supporting the development of purpose is ensuring that youth are engaged in a few potentially purposeful activities during childhood and adolescence. Potentially purposeful activities may include helping at home, volunteering in the community, participating in faith-related activities, or engaging in the arts. Empirical studies find that involvement in these kinds of pursuits typically precedes the development of purpose (Bronk 2012; Shamah 2011). Not all young people who engage in these activities will go on to develop purpose, but most youth who develop purpose report having participated in at least some of these kinds of activities early on. While it is certainly possible that young people will develop an interest in something and subsequently go out and find a way of acting on it, this is not the typical route to purpose (Bronk 2012; Damon 2008). More commonly, youth who discover purposes start out being involved in potentially purposeful activities, and over time these activities become increasingly meaningful, usually because youth find they possess a special skill or, talent, or capacity that makes them well suited to the work. Work-related and civic activities that provide youth with opportunities to take responsibility and engage in decision making are particularly likely to support the development of purpose as these activities allow youth to recognize their potential to make important contributions (Benson 2008; Shamah 2011).

It is important to note that children do not need to be exposed to expensive activities in order to discover purposes. It is not the case that parents need to enroll their children in costly music classes or private tutoring sessions. Far from it, in fact. Helping at home and volunteering in the community offer important potential avenues for the development of purpose.

That said, engaging in potentially purposeful activities early on does not lead to purpose for all youth. Presumably some youth do not find these activities to be personally meaningful, and others do not find that they possess a special talent or skill in this area. Still other youth may not find purpose in these activities because they are not encouraged to reflect on the difference their involvement in them makes. Reflection represents another important factor in the development of purpose. Youth should be encouraged to think about how their involvement impacts others in order to help them recognize how they can be useful and how they can contribute. Likewise, engaging in numerous activities is unlikely to yield a consequential experience. Rather than participating in activity after activity, youth should be encouraged to participate in fewer activities and to reflect more on the meaning derived from each one (Fry 1998).

Along these lines, discussion represents another important activity for fostering purpose. Adults should ask youth about the things that matter most to them. All too often, parents, teachers, coaches, youth leaders, and other caring adults forget to ask young people what it is they hope to accomplish in life. According to Damon (2008), initial whispers of purpose may be muted and tentative since children and adolescents may not fully grasp that they are developing a purpose. Parents and other adults can help cultivate these budding interests by encouraging young people to discuss them and by helping young people find ways of acting on them. Damon suggests that parents need not wait for these conversations to begin on their own; instead, they can start them. Thanksgiving, for instance, is a natural time to encourage youth to talk about the things they are thankful for, and "from gratitude springs not only an enhanced appreciation for our own blessings but also a desire to pass such blessing along to others- the heart and soul of purpose" (p. 141). Capitalizing on gratitude-inspiring opportunities such as the Thanksgiving holiday is likely to lead, eventually, to more valuable insights into youths' personal values and potential purposes. Through these types of conversations parents *and* youth will gain a clearer recognition of the young person's hopes, dreams, and aspirations. When adults encourage youth to discuss their aspirations, young people are better able to seriously consider what it is they hope to accomplish in life and they can begin to use this information to set priorities and make plans.

These kinds of conversations are critical to helping adults recognize youths' "sparks" (Benson 2006). According to Benson, all young people possess a "spark" or an interest that inspires them, but all too often, adults fail to recognize these things, and over time "sparks" fizzle out or languish in an under-developed form. Alarmingly, a recent study conducted at the Search Institute revealed that out of 2,000 parent-child dyads, only 26 % could identify the child's spark (Benson 2006). Clearly adults need to listen more carefully to youth and work harder to draw out the interests that inspire them. With the right support, a "spark" can serve as the foundation for a purpose. To help youth transform their "sparks," or interests, into purposes, adults should connect youth with opportunities to expand their interests and learn more about youths' plans and goals. In these conversations, it is important that adults accept what their youth are telling them and not to try to impose their own hopes or aspirations (Benson 2006; Damon 2008).

Findings from a series of recently conducted intervention studies underscore the importance of engaging youth in discussions around their personally meaningful, far horizon goals. Results suggest that discussion is not only useful for helping youth discover their purposes, but also for helping youth pursue these aims over time. For example, in one such study researchers administered purpose, goal-directedness, and life-satisfaction surveys to students at two time points roughly nine months apart during the college years (Bundick 2011). In between, a subset of these youth participated in hour-long interviews about their developing purposes. Interviews provided youth with an opportunity to articulate their aspirations, to discuss ways they planned to pursue their goals, and to reflect on the personal significance of these aims. Youth who were given the opportunity to reflect on and discuss their purposes reported higher goal-directedness and life-satisfaction scores then youth who were not given the opportunity to talk about their aspirations. The researchers (Bundick 2011) concluded that goal-directedness is a key component of purpose and that gains in life satisfaction may actually reflect an indirect increase in purpose, suggesting that the opportunity to articulate and discuss one's purpose is important to its on-going development.

A second intervention study yielded similar findings. This study assessed students' locus of control, purpose commitment, and academic achievement at two time points eighteen weeks apart (Pizzolato et al. 2011). Following the first wave of data collection, students were divided into two groups: a control group and an experimental group. The experimental group attended bi-monthly, small group meetings where a facilitator led them in discussions about their post-secondary purpose and their sense of control over their environment. The control group did not engage in any directed conversations around this topic. At time two, the experimental group showed significantly higher purpose and control scores, again suggesting that giving youth the opportunity to discuss their purposes and to reflect on their sense of efficacy, an important facet of purpose, was key to the continuing growth of purpose.

Finally, a third intervention study similarly concluded that the opportunity to consider purpose increased students' level of purposeful commitment. This study sought to determine the extent to which purpose could be cultivated among middle school students through a school-based, career education program called Make Your Work Matter (Dik et al. 2011). Make Your Work Matter is a purpose-centered intervention consisting of self-assessments of interests and skills, exploration of occupational information, and goal-setting activities all designed to address issues related to the development of purpose. Students who participated in the Make Your Work Matter counseling sessions reported a stronger sense of direction in their career choices, a clearer recognition of their interests, strengths and weaknesses, and a greater level of preparedness for the future as compared to youth who did not participate in the program. Taken together, the results of these three studies converge to suggest that the opportunity to articulate, discuss, and reflect upon the things that matter most is likely to have a significantly positive impact on the likelihood of developing and growing one's commitment to purpose over time.

Social Supports for Purpose

Parents, peers, mentors, and others can engage youth in discussions and reflections on purpose. These same individuals can also help foster purpose in other ways. One such approach is to encourage youth to embrace a long-term approach to planning and thinking in general. All too often adolescents and emerging adults find themselves overly concerned with issues that are unlikely to matter much in the future. Parents, who typically have the most contact with youth, should encourage their children to focus on ways their proximate goals align with their personally meaningful, long-term aims. This can be difficult as many adults themselves fail to focus on the long-term. This tendency persists in large part because cultural messages, especially those aimed at youth, are fixated on short horizons (Damon 2008). At times parents, teachers, and coaches are all guilty of encouraging youth to focus on short-term plans and goals, but the mass media may be the worst culprit. While it is difficult to counter the deluge of media messages, Damon argues that one way parents and other adults can encourage youth to focus on long-term aims is by discussing the things in their own lives that provide an enduring sense of purpose. Adults may derive purpose from parenting, working, volunteering, or acting on their faith, and when they share these sources of meaning with their children, they help their young people develop a critical language for purpose that allows them to keep long term aims in the front of their minds when making decisions and forming plans.

At the same time, it is also important for parents and other adults to share their personal values and beliefs with their children and adolescents. Doing so helps youth clarify their own beliefs, and personally meaningful convictions represent the very foundation of purpose (Damon 2008; Fry 1998).

Encouraging youth to view life events through a long term lens and to reflect on their aspirations are useful steps in the process of developing purpose, but they are not sufficient. Just because adolescents and emerging adults may talk about purpose does not necessarily mean they will go on to pursue one (Fry 1998). Fostering an entrepreneurial attitude in youth can help them move from talking about their deeply valued aims to acting on them (Damon 2008). An entrepreneurial attitude encompasses the ability to set clear goals and accomplish them, an optimistic, can-do outlook, persistence in the face of obstacles, tolerance for risk, resilience in the face of failure, and determination and resourcefulness to achieve measurable results. The confidence that comes from having an entrepreneurial attitude can help youth get started on their path to purpose. It can also help them stay committed over time. A purpose often represents a desire to meet a currently unaddressed social need, and pursuing such an end frequently requires youth to explore new avenues and try new things. In a study of youth with particularly strong commitments to various purposes, trailblazing was the norm (Bronk 2012). Most of the youth in the study planned to pursue novel career paths, more than half founded new organizations, and several designed their own academic majors. In each of these endeavors, an entrepreneurial attitude was essential. While these may be somewhat extreme examples, research on youth with more typical commitments similarly concludes that youth with purpose demonstrate high levels of self-efficacy (DeWitz et al. 2009; Sherer et al. 1982; Smith and Betz 2000; Solberg et al. 1993), which is a key component of an entrepreneurial attitude.

Mentor Support Parents are not the only ones who can encourage a can-do attitude among young people. Adults outside the home, including mentors, can as well. As pastors, teachers, coaches, youth leaders, and family friends, mentors are likely to be inspired by and engaged in the same activities as youth. Because they may work along side young people, they are often able to recognize talents and spot passions that may be missed by parents (Bronk 2012). Research on "sparks" suggests that young people need at least three "spark champions" or adults who can help them pursue their interests: ideally one should come from home, one from school, and one from the community (Benson 2008). These individuals can recognize the things that matter most to young people and connect youth with opportunities to pursue their personally meaningful aims.

According to Sharon Daloz Parks (2011), mentors are particularly important during the adolescent and emerging adult life stages when young people are making commitments that are likely to set them on a particular trajectory. She defines mentoring as an intentional and appropriately reciprocal relationship between two individuals, in which one is more experienced and serves as a teacher or guide to the more novice partner. In this capacity, mentors can engage in conversations where they help youth clarify their interests and aims. Once youth have identified a life purpose, mentors can recognize, support, and challenge young people's purposeful ideas (Parks 2011). While hearing from parents that they are doing well is important, adolescents and emerging adults typically seek recognition for their talents and achievements beyond the home. This recognition is critical for enhancing efficacy, self-confidence, and an entrepreneurial attitude, and mentors, because of their proximity to young people's purposeful pursuits, can be just the right people to provide that recognition. Youth with purpose report that receiving recognition and encouragement early in their involvement helped boost their initial interest and enhance their dedication (Bronk 2012). Getting involved in a new area is likely to prove difficult and at times frustrating to novices, and extrinsic rewards at this point can help keep youth motivated until their skills develop and their commitments deepen. Once this happens, external encouragement and recognition is no longer as important as purpose becomes increasingly intrinsically motivating. However, early on, recognition from others, especially highly valued mentors, may serve an important function in helping youth get started on the path to purpose.

Mentors can also offer critical support to youth in their on-going pursuit of purpose. Because they often work closely with youth around their purposes, mentors can encourage youth when they fail and offer useful guidance on how to rebound. This support can be integral to pursuing a purpose over time.

Effective mentors also challenge their protégées (Parks 2011). They may encourage youth to find novel approaches to acting on their purposes or deepening their purposeful commitments. They should also challenge youth to keep a positive attitude in spite of setbacks. Effective mentors inspire a sense of agency coupled with a sense of responsibility that can help grow youths' commitment to their aspirations. In sum, mentors can serve as an enduring source of direction, information, and reinforcement.

Youth may encounter mentors in a variety of ways. As already discussed, youth often meet adults in the natural course of pursuing their purposes (Bronk 2012). In other cases, parents and peers may introduce young people to potential mentors (Damon 2008).

Peer Support Peers can serve as another critical source of support beyond the family, especially when they share the young person's interests. Engaging in purposeful work with like-minded peers can be enjoyable, and as youth become committed to these relationships, they may also become more committed to their shared interests (Bronk 2012). While mentors are essential for the direction they can offer, like-minded peers are essential for the camaraderie they can provide. Working toward a personally meaningful aim can be difficult and frustrating at times, but being surrounded by a group of similarly-focused friends can make the job more fun thereby increasing the odds that youth stay committed over time. As young people's dedication to a purpose persists, like-minded peers can also provide an important source of emotional support and information regarding relevant resources.

Support for Purpose in Schools Beyond social support garnered from parents, mentors, and like-minded peers, ecological support can also be critical to the development of purpose. Schools, for instance, represent a potentially important context for fostering purpose (Mariano 2011; Pizzolato et al. 2011). Though it seems likely that the gains in purpose will be more lasting if the support for purpose is more enduring, empirical studies reveal that even relatively brief interventions in school settings can significantly enhance youths' purposeful commitments (e.g., Dik et al. 2011; Pizzolato et al. 2011).

A recent study designed to determine who gains most from supportive school environments revealed that students who showed some signs of developing purpose benefited more from social support associated with school settings than students who had already committed to a purpose and than students who showed little or no inclination towards developing one (Mariano et al. 2011). It makes sense that schools would have minimal impact on youth who have little or no interest in pursuing a meaningful aim, and it is also logical to conclude that support derived from school settings is not as essential to youth who have already committed to a purpose. Presumably these young people already receive support for their efforts from other sources. However, for the youth who are in the process of figuring out which aims matter most to them and sorting out how they might be able to make progress toward these aims, the support that school settings can provide is critical.

Within school settings, classrooms are an obvious place to start fostering purpose. Accordingly, researchers have proposed a variety of ways that teachers may be able to teach for purpose; however, the effectiveness of these approaches has rarely been tested. Given the benefits of purpose, broader program evaluations are warranted. Having said that, these programs have intuitive appeal, and they draw on lessons from the handful of intervention studies that have been proven to effectively boost rates of purpose among young people. Accordingly, these programs represent a promising starting point for understanding how to effectively foster purpose in the classroom.

Based on research that concludes that gains in purpose are associated with opportunities to discuss and reflect on purposeful activities (Bundick 2011; Pizzolato et al. 2011), the first approach proposes teachers make curricular modifications designed to infuse the learning experience with purpose-centered projects and discussions. Potentially effective curricular modifications vary widely but are intended to foster facets of the purpose construct. For example, history teachers could encourage students to put themselves in the place of historical leaders and to imagine how they might have handled the same situation, keeping in mind as many of the realities of the time as possible. This kind of activity is certain to foster the beyond-the-self thinking critical to the development of purpose. Similarly, science teachers might highlight moral and ethical dimensions of the work in their field. These discussions are likely to highlight students' beliefs and values, which serve as the basis of purpose. And, English teachers could select texts for students to read that highlight the search for purpose and design writing assignments that encourage students to reflect on their aspirations. Each of these lessons emphasizes important aspects of purpose.

Beyond curricular changes, teachers can also pose what Damon (2009) refers to as "the why question." Why do people study math and English? Why is it important to learn about physics? Encouraging students to focus on the significance of their lessons is not only likely to increase their motivation to work hard, but it is also likely to help focus youth on the reason behind or purpose of learning and education in general (Damon 2009). Why do we expect young people to spend nearly two decades in school? What is the point? What is the purpose? Posing this question is also likely to help students connect the aims they hope to achieve in the future with the schoolwork they are tackling at present (Van Dyke and Elias 2007), and this should make academic learning more relevant and meaningful. Moral issues pertinent to the classroom could also be discussed. Why is it wrong to cheat? Who is harmed? Teachers might even consider sharing with students their own motivations for becoming teachers. Quite often, individuals pursue this career path because they genuinely want to help students succeed, but students are all too often unaware of teachers' altruistic motivations. Addressing these kinds of questions in the classroom not only helps students better understand the purpose of education, but also exposes them to a respected adult's own quest for meaningful (Damon 2009).

A related approach to fostering purpose in the classroom focuses on employing constructivist teaching strategies. Constructivist approaches connect learning in the classroom to students' personal experiences and aspirations outside the classroom (Nash 2008). As a means of embracing constructivist teaching practices, teachers should ask students frequently what they are passionate about and listen non-judgmentally to their answers. Teachers can also engage students in conversations about their passions and in so doing help students recognize the challenges inherent in pursuing the things they care about most so they will be prepared when obstacles inevitably arise. Consistent with constructivist teaching practices, students should be encouraged to express and take pride in their voice and to take measured risks in pursuit of their aspirations (Nash 2008).

Modeling servant leadership represents yet another way teachers may be able to foster purpose in the classroom (Herman and Marlowe 2005). According to Robert Greenleaf (1998), servant leaders find ways to serve others through their position as leaders. When teachers act as servant leaders, they transform their classrooms into communities where teachers guide—rather than lead—the learning experience (Herman and Marlowe 2005). Modeling servant-leadership and setting up the classroom to inspire a sense of community is likely to empower students to assume the role of servant leaders themselves, and when they do, they will not only be building a sense of confidence to act, but also participating in a climate "in which youngsters feel genuinely concerned for one another and become involved in helping one another" (Herman and Marlowe 2005, p. 177). This lesson in thinking beyond-the-self is likely to spill over outside the classroom as youth find ways of putting their skills to work to fill personally meaningful social needs.

We can conclude that effective approaches to teaching for purpose share several features. In a variety of ways, they encourage and inspire students to consider their personal values and aspirations, how classroom learning relates to the things that matter most to them, and ways they can contribute to the broader world.

Beyond the classroom, the career counseling center represents another venue within the school where it makes sense to focus on cultivating purpose. Using a strengths-based, purpose-centered approach to helping youth consider future academic and career options helps youth make plans that reflect their personally meaningful aims and introduces youth to avenues for exploring potentially purposeful career paths (Kosine et al. 2008). This type of career counseling is designed to help youth pursue a calling, or a career that serves the greater good in a personally meaningful way.

In addition to fostering purpose in a classroom or career counseling context, school-wide efforts to support the development of purpose among students also exist. Schools are a natural context for fostering purpose for at least two significant reasons. First, the aim of schooling is to help prepare youth to become productive members of their communities (Colby et al. 2003), and the contribution inherent in purpose makes it a key component of good citizenship. Pursuing purpose, whether it is career, family, religious, or civic in nature, means working to enhance one's broader world. Accordingly, schools should foster purpose as a means of fostering citizenship, and yet few educational programs do (Koshy and Mariano 2011). Second, fostering purpose in schools is likely to increase student motivation (Damon 2009) and ultimately academic achievement. A positive relationship among purpose identification, internal locus of control, and grade point average has been found, at least among youth from lower resourced communities (Pizzolato et al. 2011).

A Colorado-based, non-profit organization called Youth Directions has designed a campus-wide curriculum designed to foster purpose among students. The organization trains teachers and administrators on how to cultivate discussions about purpose both inside and outside the classroom. The comprehensive, high school curriculum encourages youth, through classroom-based work, school-wide presentations, and a self-study component, to first, reflect on the things in their own lives about which they are particularly passionate and to consider what it is about these activities that is especially appealing. Next, youth map these appealing activity attributes onto existing career options, and eventually, they are given the opportunity to meet with and shadow professionals already doing the purposeful work they seek to do themselves. A formal evaluation of this program's effectiveness is currently underway, but key elements of the Youth Directions approach incorporate empirically established purpose-fostering strategies (e.g., Bundick 2011; Kosine et al. 2008; Pizzolato et al. 2011), and the comprehensive approach to building a culture of purpose certainly seems promising.

To this point, our discussion of educating for purpose has focused on secondary educational settings, but some colleges intentionally foster purpose, too. At these schools, professors encourage students to use their subject matter knowledge to identify and prepare for personally meaningful and socially significant careers (Cohen 1993; Cohen and Jordan 1996; Nicklin 1995). Through purpose-centered educational approaches, students engage in projects designed to connect their learning in the classroom with socially beneficial work outside the classroom. Students are encouraged to develop problem solving skills, persistence, and flexibility as a means of helping them develop the capacities required for pursing purpose.

Other colleges similarly infuse their culture with purpose by making available community service opportunities, curricula, and co-curricular activities that encourage students to discover personally meaningful, socially beneficial aims to which they can commit themselves (Braskamp et al. 2008). Building a culture of purpose requires that colleges establish shared values and a mission and identity built around purpose. Purpose-fostering college curricula are designed to instill in students a moral compass and a strong sense of responsibility. For instance, one college requires students to enroll in a seminar that helps them clarify their values, articulate their philosophy of life, and consider their conception of a good life. Infusing the college community with purpose requires offering numerous opportunities to serve the campus and the broader area. Some colleges sponsor a campus-wide day of service, during which time classes are cancelled, and students, faculty, and staff engage in a variety of service activities designed to strengthen their connection to the community. Co-curricular involvement at these schools typically centers not just on getting students engaged in multiple activities, but rather on getting students involved in fewer activities and organizations that help them more fully explore their particular interests and connect their in-class experiences with their out-of-class activities. Integrating what students learn in the classroom with what they do outside the classroom helps them identify ways of using their school-based learning to fill personally meaningful social needs.

Community Support for Purpose Clearly the home and school represent important contexts for the development of purpose, but familial and educational lessons must be reinforced by positive experiences in the broader community as well (Damon 2008). Based in part on how communities view young people, they can either foster or hinder the development of purpose. Some communities view youth as problems to be minimized, while others consider youth assets to be cultivated (Benson 2008). Communities that seek to cultivate and apply youths' strengths are more likely to support the development of purpose among their young people.

Certain kinds of communities appear more inclined than others to view youth as assets. Rural, farming communities, for example, appear to be more likely than urban and suburban communities to hold such a perspective. Because farming families in rural areas are economically tied to the land, they tend to be more socially embedded in their communities, and this can translate into greater social support for youth (Elder and Conger 2000). For example, rural adults tend to be particularly strong supporters of adolescent activities such as high school sports,

4-H, and youth-oriented religious activities, which can provide supportive contexts for youth development (Damon 2008; Elder and Conger 2000). Consistent with these findings, a recent study concluded that purpose was more prevalent among a sample of rural youth than among a similar sample of urban and suburban youth, and social support appears to be a large part of the reason why (Bronk et al., under review). This same study determined that the rural youth with the highest purpose scores also reported the highest level of perceived support from parents, peers, teachers, schools, mentors, and communities (Bronk et al., under review). Of course, social support is not exclusive to rural communities, and research finds that when youth from other types of communities feel connected to and supported by adults in their schools, they similarly report higher levels of purpose (Mariano 2011).

Religious Contexts Religious communities and activities can likewise support the development of personal aspirations. Religious faith can address fundamental questions of purpose (Francis et al. 2010; Starck 1999), and it can encourage individuals to work on behalf of personally meaningful, beyond-the-self aims, thereby inspiring purposeful acts (Emmons 2005; Fletcher 2004). Among adults, particularly devout individuals report some of the highest purpose scores (e.g., Protestant religious leaders—Crumbaugh 1968; Dominican Sisters—Crumbaugh et al. 1970), and individuals involved in religious activities, such as believing in God, (Francis 2000), praying (Francis 2000; Francis and Evans 1996; Robbins and Francis 2005), and regularly reading the bible (Francis 2000) are similarly likely to report higher purpose scores than individuals who do not engage in these activities. Additionally, being a member of a religious community has been found to predict purpose among older adults (Fletcher 2004). Interestingly, the role of religious communities in supporting the development of purpose among youth has not frequently been the topic of empirical studies. Given that many youth are involved in these programs and that religious contexts are strongly associated with increased purpose levels among adults, this represents a worthwhile line of inquiry.

Therapeutic Support for Purpose While most individuals who discover purpose do so in the course of their daily lives, some individuals struggle to find meaning and consequently turn to counseling. Logotherapy, introduced by Viktor Frankl (1959), is a therapeutic approach that helps individuals discover their life's purpose. It applies the principles of existential philosophy to clinical practice (Crumbaugh and Maholick 1964). At Logotherapy's core is a belief that humanity's primary motivational force is a "will to meaning," and logotherapists help patients discover the meaning in their lives in an effort to relieve symptoms of purposelessness including boredom, depression, and anxiety. According to Frankl (1984), people can discover purpose by creating a work, completing a deed, enduring a challenging experience, or interacting with others in meaningful ways that benefit the broader world. Frankl believed that even people in dive circumstances could discover purpose by rising above the situation. It is always possible, Frankt Argued for, individuals to "turn a personal tragedy into triumph" (Frankl 1984, p. 170) As a concentration camp inmate, Frankl managed to do this himself.

Logoanalysis represents another style of therapy based on the same principles as logotherapy, but it is delivered through Socratic dialogue as opposed to a more traditional clinical approach. Like logotherapy, logoanalysis seeks to aid people in discovering the hidden meaning in their lives (Crumbaugh and Henrion 2001; Crumbaugh and Maholick 1964). To do this, therapists help individuals focus on the positives in their lives, rather than dwelling on the negatives (Crumbaugh and Henrion 2001). Therapists also help patients identify and clarify personally significant values and beliefs as these form an important basis for purpose development.

Beyond receiving support for purpose in one-on-one counseling sessions, individuals can also utilize self-help options. For example, Joseph Fabry (1980, 1988), the past Director of the Logotherapy Institute and a close friend and disciple of Viktor Frankl's, designed a self-help book based on Frankl's therapeutic approach. The self-study course presents individuals with a series of exercises and activities designed to help them discover a purpose for their lives. Fabry believed people needed to develop certain capacities in orders discover their purpose. For instance, he recognized that purpose and identity were closely intertwined, and accordingly, his workbook underscores the importance of developing a deep sense of self-understanding as a first step to developing purpose. Fabry also believed that individuals seeking purpose needed to be able to see alternatives in the world around them. His book encourages individuals to recognize that circumstances can get better and to focus on ways that they can contribute to bringing about improvement. Coupled with this, the workbook includes a series of activities designed to help individuals take personal responsibility for applying their special talents to address social needs. Finally, Fabry encourages purpose-seekers to reach beyond their own egocentricity and toward others in order to develop a meaningful life purpose. Other self-help books and personal coaching programs designed to foster purpose exist, but most lack a strong theoretical foundation. Accordingly, they are not discussed here.

A variety of therapeutic approaches to helping people find purpose. Exist workbook activities and exercises, counseling, and Socratic dialogue have all been employed in this pursuit. Most people do not seek professional help to discover purpose; however, elements of the practices outlined here could be effectively applied by parents, teachers, mentors, and others to help individuals discover and pursue purpose in their own lives.

It is clear from this discussion that effective approaches to fostering purpose share key features. For instance, they highlight the importance of offering individuals the opportunity to engage in potentially purposeful activities and of providing a high degree of support throughout the discovery and commitment phases. Effective programs, interventions, and approaches also feature a long term focus. While a small body of research reveals that even relatively short term interventions can significantly increase rates of purpose (Bundick 2011; Pizzolato et al. 2011), other studies conclude that on-going support is more likely than short term interventions to lead to a more enduring commitment (Bronk 2012; Koshy and Mariano 2011). Also, effective approaches encourage, in some form, purpose-driven discussions (Koshy and Mariano 2011), which provide youth with a platform for articulating their aims and expanding their knowledge of the things that matter most to them.

Having these conversations with parents, teachers, mentors, and peers can help youth thoughtfully consider what it is they hope to accomplish and how they plan to go about doing so. Additionally, these discussions, especially early in the process of discovering personal aspirations, should focus on identifying personal values and beliefs, which serve as the foundation of purpose (Damon 2008). Next, reflection is vital (Bundick 2011). Youth should be encouraged to reflect on their personally meaningful goals and to consider ways they can apply their particular character strengths and talents to make progress toward meaningful aims. Finally, youth should be engaged. To support the development of purpose, youth should be active in service-learning opportunities, meaningful paid work, apprenticeships, and other roles where they can be empowered to make decisions, develop a sense of efficacy, and be inspired by a potential purpose.

Despite the fairly lengthy discussion in this chapter, there is still much to be learned about how a stable and enduring sense of purpose emerges from formative experiences and how people and contexts can best foster the development of personal aspirations. Much of the research presented in this chapter is theoretical, and as such, it needs to be tested. Much of it centers on ways of fostering purpose in family and school settings, but what can be done to support the development of purpose in other key settings, including religious and extra-curricular ones? We know that youth who feel supported by and connected to their communities are more likely than youth who do not to report purposes in their lives (Bronk et al., under review), but we do not know exactly why. What is happening for these youth that leads them to develop and pursue purpose? Further, in addition to examining the role of positive experiences, such as familial and community support, the role of negative experiences should also be explored. Frankl (1959) believed that his own purpose in life not only sustained him during the incredibly difficult experience of being held in a concentration camp, but that it also became clearer to him as a result of these difficult circumstances. In spite of this, little empirical work has focused on the role of negative experiences in fostering purpose.

Finally, how are different types of purposes supported? Do the same strategies effectively foster religious, familial, and civic purposes, or are different types of support required for different forms of purpose? The following chapter will take up this question and will focus more directly on empirical research conducted on different types of purposes.

References

Benson, P. L. (2006). *All kids are our kids: What communities must do to raise caring and responsible children and adolescents* (2nd ed.) San Francisco: Jossey-Bass.

Benson, P. L. (2008). *Sparks: How parents can help ignite the hidden strengths of teenagers*. San Francisco: Jossey Bass.

Boyd, B. (2009). Purpose-driven life. *American Scholar, 78*(2), 24–34.

Braskamp, L., Trautvetter, L. C., & Ward, K. (2008). Putting students first: Promoting lives of purpose and meaning. *About Campus, 13*(1), 26–32.

Bronk, K. C. (2012). A grounded theory of youth purpose. *Journal of Adolescent Research, 27,* 78–109. http://dx.doi.org/10.1177/0743558411412958.
Bronk, K. C., Finch, W. H., & Talib, T. (2010). Purpose among high ability adolescents. *High Ability Studies, 21*(2), 133–145.
Bronk, K. C., Finch, W. H., Youngs, A., & Kollman, J. (under review). *The development of rural youth purpose.*
Bronk, K. C., Hill, P., Lapsley, D., Talib, T., & Finch, W. H. (2009). Purpose, hope, and life satisfaction in three age groups. *Journal of Positive Psychology, 4*(6), 500–510.
Bundick, M. (2011). The benefits of reflecting on and discussing purpose in life in emerging adulthood. *New Directions for Youth Development, 132,* 89–103.
Cohen, A. (1993). A new educational paradigm. *Phi Delta Kappan, 74*(10), 791–795.
Cohen, A., & Jordan, J. (1996). Audrey Cohen College System of Education: Purpose-centered education. In S. Stringfield, S. M. Ross, & L. Smith (Eds.), *Bold plans for school restructuring: The New American Schools designs* (pp. 25–52). Mahwah, NJ: Erlbaum.
Colby, A., Ehrlich, T., Beaumont, E., Stephens, J., & Shulman, L. (2003). *Educating citizens: Preparing America's undergraduates for lives of moral and civic responsibility.* San Francisco: Jossey Bass/ Carnegie Foundation for the Advancement of Teaching.
Crumbaugh, J. C. (1968). Cross-validation of purpose in life test based on Frankl's concepts. *Journal of Individual Psychology, 24*(1), 74–81.
Crumbaugh, J. C., & Henrion, R. (2001). How to find meaning and purpose in life for the third millennium. *The International Forum for Logotherapy, 24,* 1–9.
Crumbaugh, J. C., & Maholick, L. T. (1964). An experimental study in existentialism: The psychometric approach to Frankl's concept of noogenic neurosis. *Journal of Clinical Psychology, 20*(2), 200–207.
Crumbaugh, J. C., Raphael, S. M., & Shrader, R. R. (1970). Frankl's will to meaning in a religious order. *Journal of Clinical Psychology, 26,* 206–7.
Damon, W. (2008). *The path to purpose: Helping our children find their calling in life.* New York: Free Press.
Damon, W. (2009). The why question: Teachers can instill a sense of purpose. *Education Next, 9*(3), 84.
DeWitz, S. J., Woolsey, M. L., & Walsh, B. W. (2009). College student retention: An exploration of the relationship between self-efficacy beliefs and purpose in life among college students. *Journal of College Student Development, 50*(1), 19–34.
Dik, B. J., Steger, M. F., Gibson, A., & Peisner, W. (2011). Make your work matter: Development and pilot evaluations of a purpose-centered career education intervention. *New Directions for Youth Development, 132,* 59–73.
Elder, G. H., & Conger, R. D. (2000). *Children of the land: Adversity and success in rural America.* Chicago: University of Chicago Press.
Emmons, R. A. (2005). Striving for the sacred: Personal goals, life meaning, and religion. *Journal of Social Issues, 61,* 731–746.
Fabry, J. (1980). *The pursuit of meaning: Viktor Frankl, Logotherapy, and life.* New York: HarperCollins Publishers.
Fabry, J. (1988). *Guideposts to meaning: Discovering what really matters.* Oakland, CA: Harbinger Publications.
Fletcher, S. K. (2004). Religion and life meaning: Differentiating between religious beliefs and religious community in constructing life meaning. *Journal of Aging Studies, 18,* 171–185.
Francis, L. J. (2000). The relationship between bible reading and purpose in life among 13–15-year olds. *Mental Health, Religion, & Culture, 3*(1), 27–36.
Francis, L. J., & Evans, T. E. (1996). The relationship between personal prayer and purpose in life among churchgoing and non-churchgoing 12–15 year olds in the UK. *Religious Education, 91,* 9–21.
Francis, L. J., Jewell, A., & Robbins, M. (2010). The relationship between religious orientation, personality, and purpose in life among an older Methodist sample. *Mental Health, Religion & Culture, 13*(7–8), 777–791.

Frankl, V. (1959). *Man's search for meaning*. New York: Simon & Schuster.
Frankl, V. (1984). *Man's search for meaning: Revised and updated*. New York: Simon & Schuster.
Fry, P. A. (1998). The development of personal meaning and wisdom in adolescence: A reexamination of moderating and consolidating factors and influences. In P. T. P. Wong (Ed.), *The human quest for meaning: A handbook of psychological research and clinical applications* (2nd ed., pp. 91–110). New York: Routledge.
Greenleaf, R. K. (1998). *The power of servant-leadership*. San Francisco: Berrett-Koehler Publishers.
Herman, D. V., & Marlowe, M. (2005). Modeling meaning in life: The teacher as servant leader. *Reclaiming Children and Youth, 14*(3), 175–178.
Ishida, R., & Okada, M. (2006). Effects of a firm purpose in life on anxiety and sympathetic nervous activity caused by emotional stress: Assessment by psychological method. *Stress and health: Journal of the International Society for the Investigation of Stress, 22*(4), 275–281.
Klinger, K. (1998). The search for meaning in evolutionary perspective. (pp. 27–50). In P. T. P. Wong, & P. S. Fry (Eds.), *The human quest for meaning*. Mahwah, NJ: Lawrence Erlbaum Associates.
Koshy, S. I., & Mariano, J. M. (2011). Promoting youth purpose: A review of the literature. *New Directions for Youth Development, 132*, 13–29.
Kosine, N., Steger, M. F., & Duncan, S. (2008). Purpose-centered career development: A strengths-based approach to finding meaning and purpose in careers. *Professional School Counseling, 12*(2), 133–136.
Mariano, J. M., Going, J., Schrock, K., & Sweeting, K. (2011). Youth purpose and perceived social supports among ethnic minority middle school girls. *Journal of Youth Studies, 14*(8), 921–938.
Mariano, J. M., & Vaillant, G. E. (2012). Purpose among the "Greatest Generation." *Journal of Positive Psychology*. doi:10.1080/17439760.2012.686624.
Moran, S. (2009). Purpose: Giftedness in intrapersonal intelligence. *High Ability Studies, 20*(2), 143–159. doi:10.1080/13598130903358501..
Nanay, B. (2010). Group selection and our obsession with the meaning of life. *The Monist, 93*(1), 76–95.
Nash, R. J. (2008). A personal reflection on educating for meaning. *About Campus, 13*(2), 17–24.
Nicklin, J. L. (1995, July 14). Education with a purpose. *Chronicle of Higher Education, 41*(44), A13–A14.
Parks, S. D. (2011). *Big questions, worthy dreams: Mentoring emerging adults in their search for meaning, purpose, and faith (revised ed)*. San Francisco: Jossey Bass.
Pizzolato, J. E., Brown, E. L., & Kanny, M. A. (2011). Purpose plus: Supporting youth purpose, control, and academic achievement. *New Directions for Youth Development, 132*, 75–88.
Robbins, M., & Francis, L. J. (2005). Purpose in life and prayer among Catholic and Protestant adolescents in Northern Ireland. *Journal of Research on Christian Education, 14*(1), 73–93.
Shamah, D. (2011). Supporting a strong sense of purpose: Lessons from a rural community. *New Directions for Youth Development, 132*, 45–58.
Sherer, M., Maddux, J. E., Mercandante, B., Prentice-Dunn, S., Jacobs, B., & Rogers, R. W. (1982). The Self-Efficacy Scale: Construction and validation. *Psychological Reports, 51*, 663–671.
Smith, H., & Betz, N. E. (2000). Development and evaluation of a measure of social self-efficacy in college students. *Journal of Career Assessment, 8*, 282–302.
Solberg, V. S., O'Brien, K., Villareal, P., Kennel, R., & Davis, B. J. (1993). Self-efficacy and Hispanic college students: Validation of the college self-efficacy instrument. *Hispanic Journal of Behavioral Sciences, 15*, 80–95.
Starck, P. L. (1999). Micro foundations of religion: A revised theory. *Sociological Theory, 17*(3), 264–289.
VanDyke, C. J., & Elias, M. J. (2007). How forgiveness, purpose, and religiosity are related to the mental health and well-being of youth. *Mental Health, Religion, & Culture*, 10(4), 395–415.

Chapter 6
Inspiring Types of Purpose

A purpose represents a *generalized* commitment to engage in a meaningful way with the world beyond-the-self (emphasis added; Damon 2008; Damon et al. 2003). Accordingly, purpose is diffuse and influences many aspects of life, likely including career, hobby, and familial choices. In fact, a purpose can be so broad that it composes a central component of one's sense of identity (Bronk 2011; Damon 2008; Erikson 1968). Chapter 4 (Purpose across the Lifespan) features a more complete discussion of the relationship between purpose and identity, but briefly, for individuals with purpose, their sense of identity is largely intertwined with their personally meaningful aims. Put another way, who they are and who they hope to become is significantly influenced by what they hope to accomplish in life (Bronk 2011). For that reason, a person who finds purpose in helping others may choose to pursue a career as a physician where she can serve her patients, have a family where she can help her children become productive citizens, and be active in church where she can volunteer at the local food bank. This fictitious person's purpose focuses on helping others, but her valued aim manifests itself through her career, her family, and her religious and community commitments. Categorizing a purpose as diffuse as this is a challenge. It could be argued that this individual simultaneously demonstrates religious, familial, career, and community-oriented purposes in life. In spite of the difficulty in classifying aspirations, however, it is important to know what kinds of aims inspire individuals in order to effectively foster the development of purpose. It is also important to learn more about the developmental trajectory and supports required for different types of purposes, since these are likely to vary. Therefore, in spite of the difficulty involved in categorizing purposes, doing so represents a useful endeavor.

In attempting to do this, it is important to keep in mind the distinction between purpose and purposeful engagement. Whereas purpose represents the personally meaningful aim one is working toward, purposeful engagement represents the way one makes progress toward this aim. In other words, purpose is the *end* toward which one aspires, and purposeful engagement is the *means* through which one progresses toward that end. To determine what the "end" is, interviews are useful. Participants should be repeatedly asked why they are doing the things they are doing. Their ultimate "why" typically reveals their purpose. Accordingly, in the example

K. C. Bronk, *Purpose in Life*, DOI 10.1007/978-94-007-7491-9_6,

above, if the woman said she sought to help others because it seemed like the right thing to do, then her purpose would be categorized most accurately as an altruistic personal value. However, if she noted that helping others was important because she believed it was what God called her to do, then her purpose would best be classified as a religious aim. And, if the reason she gave for wanting to help others was because this was the most efficient way of contributing to her local community, then her purpose would be categorized as a community or civic-oriented aspiration. As this example illustrates, classifying purpose is a complex process and it is only possible when individuals are given the chance to explain why the aims they seek hold personal significance.

Unfortunately, few studies of purpose offer participants the opportunity to expand on the reasons behind their hopes and plans. What is more, few existing studies even distinguish between purpose and purposeful engagement. In some cases researchers themselves fail to make this distinction, and in other cases researchers allow lay people to identify the sources of their own purpose, leaving open the possibility that they will generate sources of purposeful engagement rather than sources of purpose.

One reason individuals—researchers and lay people alike—confuse purpose with purposeful engagement is because it is easier to talk about what we are doing than it is to discuss why we are doing it. In the hundreds of interviews my colleagues and I have conducted with adolescents and emerging adults, we consistently find that individuals discuss their goals eloquently and in great detail. Young people are expected to have goals, and as such, they tend to be readily accessible for discussion. But when asked why they are pursuing these goals—what it is that they ultimately hope to achieve—we often get blank stares, at least at first. Giving participants time and offering them prompts can help them verbalize not only what they hope to accomplish, but also the reason they hope to achieve these aims.

While articulating one's purpose may be a challenge, it is typically one adolescents and emerging adults enjoy undertaking. Interview participants tend to appreciate the opportunity to reflect on why they are doing the things they are doing and why they aspire to the goals to which they aspire. High school and college interviewees regularly thank us for the opportunity to participate in purpose interviews. They express gratitude for the rare opportunity to reflect on the things that matter most to them.

Given this, it is particularly surprising that we, as parents, teachers, and adults concerned about the well-being of young people, do not offer adolescents and emerging adults this opportunity more regularly. In fact, there are virtually no structured opportunities for youth to reflect on their ultimate aims. College applications represent one interesting exception, for at least some young people. Most applications ask youth to include a "statement of purpose" of sorts, and many young people struggle to articulate this. Perhaps if we encouraged youth to consider and discuss their purposes sooner and more regularly, this task would not be so daunting.

Because purpose is so diffuse and because it can be difficult to disentangle from purposeful engagement, research focused directly on categorizing different kinds of purposes has not been highly reliable. There are however, other bodies of research that shed light on likely categories of personally meaningful aspirations. Philosophers, for example, frequently consider potential sources of purpose and meaning. Robert Nozick (1989) suggested that creating, parenting, and loving represented potentially purposeful activities. Interestingly, consistent with the definition of purpose, each of these sources represents a form of doing or being actively engaged. Bertrand Russell was another philosopher who contemplated sources of purpose, and he argued that individuals often meaningfully invest their energy in families, work, and personal interests (as cited in Ryff and Singer 1998). These examples underscore the important beyond-the-self aspect of purpose.

Reviewing research on the different sources of meaning in life is also useful for discerning potential types of purposes, and in some cases forms of purposeful engagement. Empirical studies of categories of meaning can inform our understanding of the aims to which people aspire.

Before delving into this body of research, however, it is important to bear in mind the distinction between meaning and purpose. As discussed in greater detail in Chap. 1 (Introduction and Definition), purpose represents a stable and generalized *intention* to accomplish something that is at once meaningful to the self and at the same time leads to productive engagement *with some aspect of the world beyond-the-self* (emphasis added; Damon 2008; Damon et al. 2003). In other words, for something to comprise a purpose in life it must constitute a far-horizon aim to impact the broader world in some personally meaningful way. Meaning, on the other hand, represents a broader array of goals and interests. People may find meaning in aims that are both other-oriented (e.g., helping others) and purely self-oriented (e.g., becoming wealthy). Further, sources of meaning need not be goal-oriented at all, since anything that makes one's life more personally significant can be said to be meaningful. As such, having good health may be meaningful, but it is not necessarily goal oriented nor does it necessarily involve a beyond-the-self concern. Accordingly, it does not represent a form of purpose. However, helping others to preserve their good health may provide purpose.

Because meaning is a broad concept without many qualifiers, it tends to be more accessible than purpose, and, not surprisingly, sources of meaning have been researched with greater regularity than sources of purpose. In fact, a moderately large body of empirical research on sources of meaning exists, and this literature points to some potential sources of purpose and purposeful engagement.

A team of researchers, interested in identifying the most commonly cited sources of personal meaning, asked participants to complete the Meaning Essay Document. This tool asks adolescent (DeVogler and Ebersole 1983), emerging adult (DeVogler and Ebersole 1980), and adult (DeVogler and Ebersole 1981) participants "to write about, rank in order, and give an example of the three strongest meanings in their life" (DeVogler and Ebersole 1981, p. 88). None of the categories that emerged represent aims, so none point to potential sources of purpose, but several of the categories highlight a commitment to activities, and accordingly illuminate potential sources of purposeful engagement. These categories include the following: having relationships (an interpersonal orientation including family, friends, and romantic partners), holding beliefs (living according to one's religious, political or social beliefs), participating in service (helping or serving others), and carrying out one's life work (derived from an occupation or job; DeVogler and Ebersole 1981; Ebersole 1998). These categories represent *potential* sources of purposeful engagement, rather than *actual* sources of purposeful engagement, because we need to know more about why each category is personally meaningful to determine if it represents a form of genuine purposeful engagement. For instance, we cannot know for sure if a category such as "relationships" represents a form of purposeful engagement without knowing more about why relationships are personally significant. If people find meaning in relationships primarily because of what being in a relationship can do for them, then this likely is not a source of purpose, but if they find meaning in relationships at least in part because of what they allow them to do for others, then it likely does represent a source of purposeful engagement. Other sources of meaning (e.g., health, obtaining, pleasure, appearance, and growth) emerged from this line of inquiry as well, but they were either exclusively self-oriented or lacked even a potential goal orientation, and as such they do not shed light on potential forms of purpose.

Another team of researchers, using the Sources of Meaning Profile (SOMP; Prager 1996), identified sources of meaning among Australian and Canadian adults. Again, only those results that could potentially represent sources of purpose are discussed here. The categories of meaning that emerged included: supporting personal relationships, participating in hobbies, and preserving values and ideals. These categories *could* represent beyond-the-self goals, and so they *could* represent sources of purpose, but again, we need to know why each is personally significant to know for sure.

Using the related Personal Meaning Profile (PMP; Wong 1998), which was designed to uncover sources of meaning in life, (and is discussed in greater detail in Chap. 2, Measuring Purpose), two teams of researchers concluded that religion, relationships, self-transcendence, and fair treatment represented commonly cited sources of meaning among adults (Wong and Fry 1998) and adolescents (Rathi and Rastogi 2007). Interestingly, the Personal Meaning Profile asks participants to envision their ideally meaningful life, and hedonic pursuits did not emerge as an important component of this, suggesting that the beyond-the-self component of purpose is not only significant, but also that it may be consistent with adults' conceptions of personal meaningfulness (Wong and Fry 1998).

In yet another study designed to determine sources of meaning, participants actually completed the Purpose in Life test (PIL; Crumbauagh and Maholick 1964) and took part in interviews about the "meaningful events" in their lives (Baum and Stewart 1990). Researchers categorized participants' responses into the following categories of potentially purposeful engagement: pursuing careers, supporting relationships, and engaging in independent pursuits.

It is interesting to note that despite the many different instruments administered to assess sources of meaning, the results are fairly consistent. Relationships, careers, hobbies, and personal values and beliefs represent the most consistent sources of meaning, and potentially the most common sources of purpose and purposeful engagement, too.

Taken together, research on meaning coupled with philosophers' theories on ways people are likely to be purposefully engaged suggests that purpose is derived from and manifested through engagement in families, religion, careers, artistic pursuits, and civic activities. Some empirical research has been conducted on each of these categories of purpose, but the vast majority of the research has focused on religious and spiritual avenues for purpose and purposeful engagement. Included, along with the discussion of religious purpose and other forms of purpose and purposeful engagement that follow, are brief case studies of individuals who exemplify each of the different types of purpose. These case studies are included to illustrate what these types of purpose look like in real life and to further demonstrate the challenge inherent in categorizing purpose since several of them could provide examples of more than one type of personally meaningful aspiration. The case studies were drawn from two different longitudinal studies: one is a five-year study of youth with particularly intense commitments to various purposes (Bronk 2005, 2011, 2012) and the other is a one-year longitudinal study of more typical forms of purpose among rural youth (Bronk et al., under review). Because the vast majority of research on types of purpose focuses on religious aims, this category of purpose is discussed first.

Religious Purposes

Purpose is central to the very essence of faith (Tillich 1952), and in a variety of ways, religion can serve as an important source of purpose and as a significant avenue for purposeful engagement (Sommer et al. 2012). This may seem obvious, but in fact there is no uniform way in which religious experiences are likely to foster or frame an individual's sense of purpose (Van Dyke and Elias 2007). One way religion may inspire purpose is by addressing existential questions of the larger meaning of life. The teachings and rituals inherent in most religions explicitly address fundamental questions of meaning and purpose (Francis et al. 2010; Starck 1999). Another way religion may support the development of purpose is by encouraging individuals to focus on themselves in relation to God. In so doing, individuals can gain a greater understanding of their "sacred selves," and this process can help them transcend their secular lives (George 2000, p. 26). By encouraging a beyond-the-self focus with regards to developing personally meaningful aims, religious instruction is likely to foster purpose. Lastly, religion may inspire purpose by providing a meaningful framework for people's lives. The quest for spiritual salvation and a life lived in accord with God's wishes can help put life events into a comprehensible context. Religion can serve as an important source of purpose by investing human existence with meaning through the establishment of goals and value systems that pertain to all aspects of an individual's life (Emmons 2005). Put otherwise, religion can provide people with a vision of what they should be striving for (Pargament and Park 1995). In each of these ways, religion can serve as a significant resource for the discovery and pursuit of purpose (Fletcher 2004).

In the latter view, religion is viewed through a goal-framework. While we may not typically identify religion as a goal, some have argued that goal pursuit is central to faith, and that a goal framework allows for a fuller understanding of the relationship between religion and purpose in life (Emmons 2005). Seeking to serve God, to unite with God, and to live according to God's will represent long-term aims that can provide individuals with important source of motivation that guide their daily behavior and shape their long-term plans. Given that a purpose also represents a personally meaningful, long-term aim, this goal-oriented perspective on religion overlaps with purpose. As an aim, faith represents not a separate, compartmentalized dimension of life, but instead an orientation to the world that guides the whole person and provides direction to significant goals and strivings (Emmons 2005; Fowler 1981). Some people's religious convictions are so all-encompassing that they comprise a central part of their sense of identity (Dillon 1999), similar to purpose (Bronk 2011; Damon 2008; Erikson 1968, 1980). Both religious and purposeful beliefs can represent aspects of identity and can frame the pursuit of personally meaningful goals (Bronk 2011; Emmons 1999; Tirri and Quinn 2010).

"Spiritual strivings" (Emmons 2005) and purpose also overlap around the type of long-term aims they inspire. Both purposeful and religious aims are transcendent in nature. Accordingly, they represent personally meaningful goals that serve an aim larger than the self. Goal-oriented engagement in religious purpose can take many forms, including martyrdom, helping the poor, converting non-believers, being used by God, seeking to serve others, and treating others well in the quest for eternal life (Emmons 2005).

Clearly religion and purpose represent related constructs, but what does the relationship between them look like in practice? Based on interview and surveys conducted with a small sample of young people with clear purposes, in life researchers (Mariano and Damon 2008) proposed five, empirically based, working models of the association. The first model suggests that religious beliefs can help people determine that they want to contribute, which can eventually lead to purpose. In this view, the desire to work toward beyond-the-self aims may derive from spiritual convictions. The second model proposes that religious beliefs can infuse personal goals with meaning that they might otherwise lack. Doing one's job, for instance, may take on greater significance when viewed through a religious lens. The third and fourth models point out that religious beliefs and religious communities can offer individuals developing purpose a critical source of support. Spiritual communities often encourage and share purposeful and religious aims. Finally, the fifth model represents the integration of religious beliefs and purpose. According to this model, purpose and religious beliefs can be synonymous; for some individuals, their purposes *are* their religious aims.

Given that purpose is so central to religion it is not surprising that studies consistently find that purpose and faith are positively related among both adolescents (Crandall and Rasmussen 1975; Francis and Burton 1994; Soderstrom and Wright 1977) and adults (Chamberlain and Zika 1988). Nor is it surprising to find that particularly devout individuals report some of the highest purpose scores (e.g., Protestant religious leaders—Crumbaugh 1968; Dominican Sisters—Crumbaugh et al. 1970) or that individuals engaged in religious activities, such as personal prayer (Francis 2000; Francis and Evans 1996; Robbins and Francis 2005), believing in God (Francis 2000), and reading the Bible regularly (Francis 2000), report higher rates of purpose then individuals who do not engage in these activities.

Individuals who find purpose in faith reap many benefits. For example, health benefits include improved immune function, reduced levels of depression, lower blood pressure, and delayed mortality (Townsend et al. 2000). And, social benefits include increased satisfaction with relationships (Mahoney et al. 1999) and a lower rate of divorce (Booth et al. 1995; Clydesdale 1997). Individuals who find purpose in religion are also likely to navigate the aging process more successfully (Koenig et al. 1988) and to experience greater levels of psychological well-being (Robins and Francis 2000).

Religious individuals also report higher levels of subjective well-being as compared to non-religious individuals, but this relationship only holds when they also report a high level of purpose (French and Joseph 1999). Similarly, purpose has been found to mediate the relationship between religiosity and life satisfaction and between religious behaviors and well-being (Steger and Frazier 2005). We can conclude from these studies that pursing a religious purpose confers important physical and psychological health benefits.

Nature and Quality of Religious Commitment While religion can represent an important source of purpose, researchers have found that the nature and quality of religious commitments influence the degree to which religion and purpose are likely to be related. People conceive of faith in different ways and to varying degrees. They also commit to religious beliefs for different reasons. Empirical studies find that individuals' conceptions of and orientations to religion influence the level of their commitment to purpose. For instance, some people orient to faith from a quest perspective. People with a quest orientation (Batson and Ventis 1982) tend to approach religion in a way that acknowledges that they do not know—and likely never will know—the truth about religious matters. They deem religious questions as important and they seek answers to them, but they do so knowing that they are unlikely to ever solve the mystery of faith. Other people espouse either extrinsic or intrinsic orientations to religion (Allport and Ross 1967). Individuals with extrinsic religious orientations tend to use religion for their own means, including for security, solace, social outlets, status, or power. Individuals with intrinsic religious orientations view faith as their "master motive" (Allport and Ross 1967, p. 434). For them, all other aims are subordinated to their religious goals. Individuals who are intrinsically oriented to faith strive to live according to their religious beliefs.

Studies reveal that purpose is significantly related to an intrinsic orientation to religion (Byrd et al. 2007; Crandall and Rasmussen 1975; Paloutzian and Ellison 1982; Soderstrom and Wright 1977). Consistent with this finding, researchers (Crandall and Rasmussen 1975) have also determined that individuals who attribute greater importance to the value of salvation score higher on purpose than individuals who favor values such as pleasure, excitement, or comfort. In this way the nature of one's orientation to faith can impact the association between religious commitment and purpose.

The certainty of one's faith can similarly influence the nature of religious purpose. An empirical study with an older adult sample found that participants could be segmented based on the degree of certainty in their religious convictions (Fletcher 2004). Individuals were categorized into one of three groups, including believers, belongers, and doubters. These designations bear some resemblance to the intrinsic, extrinsic, and quest orientations to religion, respectively. Believers seek to do whatever it is they believe God wants them to do. They typically find purpose in serving God or in being used by God for his purposes. Belongers derive meaning through serving others and in so doing hope to achieve God's approval. Finally, doubters do not derive meaning from their belief in God at all. Instead they seek to help others and leave behind a meaningful legacy. While believers find purpose in their relationship with God, belongers and doubters tend to find meaning through their social interactions with others, including those in their religious communities. In this manner, the level of certainty in religious beliefs can impact the way individuals derive purpose from them.

Another way that individuals differ in terms of the nature of their religious convictions has to do with the content of their beliefs, and this too can influence the likelihood that individuals will commit to a purpose. Individuals can have a committed or consensual relationship to faith (Allen and Spilka 1967). Committed individuals tend to have belief systems that are abstract, discerning, well differentiated, flexible and open, and relevant to their lives. Individuals with a consensual orientation tend to have belief systems that are concrete, literal, vague, simplistic, and undifferentiated, inflexible, and detached. Committed orientations to religion are associated with higher rates of life purpose (Soderstrom and Wright 1977).

Lastly, the depth of one's religious beliefs can also influence the likelihood of developing a religious a purpose in life. Davidson (1972) proposed a model that categorized individuals along two dimensions: one that reflects the depth of one's religious commitment, or commitment to God, and another that assesses one's moral commitment to others. True believers are characterized by strong moral and spiritual commitments, mainliners by moderate moral and spiritual commitment, and unbelievers by generally weak moral and spiritual commitments. Humanists demonstrate strong moral but weak spiritual commitments, and fundamentalists demonstrate weak moral but strong spiritual commitments. True believers report significantly higher purpose scores than other individuals (Soderstrom and Wright 1977). Taken together this body of research finds that religious purpose is most prevalent among true believers with mature religious commitments (Soderstrom and Wright 1977).

Periods of Increased Prevalence of Religious Purpose Religiosity increases with age (Courtenay et al. 1992), and accordingly, while religious purposes are prevalent across the lifespan, they are particularly common among older adults (Fletcher 2004). As discussed in greater length in Chap. 4 (Purpose across the Lifespan), older adults often suffer from the "structural lag problem," (Riley et al. 1994) whereby opportunities and roles for purposeful engagement begin to evaporate as individuals approach late adulthood (Ryff and Singer 2008). Coupled with this is the reality that death is drawing near, and this realization often inspires increased religious devotion. These realities likely contribute to the particularly high prevalence, of religious purposes among later adults (Fletcher 2004).

Another time that religious purposes appear to be particularly prevalent is immediately following conversion. Converts to a new faith report significantly higher purpose scores within a week of conversion than non-convert controls (Paloutzian 1981). A month later converts' purpose scores tend to drop. This suggests that a sense of purpose, while an enduring aspect of the self, does increase and decrease, at least to some degree, depending on life events. A fuller discussion of the state-like and trait-like qualities of the life purpose construct is included in Chap. 4 (Purpose across the Lifespan).

Case Study of Religious Purpose Following is a brief picture of an adolescent, interviewed three times over a five-year study of purpose, who demonstrates clear signs of religious purpose (Bronk 2011, 2012; Damon 2008). Marta[1], a Latina living in Northern California, was 18-years-old when she was first interviewed. A senior in high school, she was passionate about her religious faith, and described herself first and foremost as a "Christian." She had attended a private, Christian school since she was 10-years-old and was active in her church, where she was a member of the worship team, played the keyboard, and sang in weekly services. When Marta was 8-years-old, she was "born again" in Christ. Throughout her childhood, she attended church regularly with her Dad, but she said she did not really know what it all meant until she got older. As an adolescent, she began to reflect more deeply on her faith and meditate daily on scriptures. At her Quinceanera, a traditional Hispanic coming of age celebration for girls on their fifteenth birthdays, her pastor told her that God was calling her to serve low-income Hispanics living in the United States and abroad by pursuing a career in medicine. Marta believed the prophecy, as she had felt called to do the same thing. In spite of the fact that no one in her family had attended college before, Marta spent her summers working in a medical lab at a local university and applied to college.

When we interviewed Marta two years later, she was busier than before, but her faith was still strong and her plan to pursue a career in medicine remained intact. She was putting herself through a highly competitive 4-year college and working toward a pre-med degree. Two more years later, Marta had graduated from college and was busy working in a hospital trying to pay off her school loans while she decided which branch of medicine to pursue. At this point in her life, Marta was not as active in her church community, but her religious faith was still strong. "[God's] been really good to me. I honestly don't think I would have made it through [college] if it wasn't for His grace all the time, like with my teachers, my grades, and everything. I barely made it through a lot of classes, honestly. Like science classes at [my college]- wow- especially when you're working, so it was really—He's been taking care of me ever since then."

Marta's story provides a useful picture of what religious purpose looks like in real life. Her aim, to serve God, was personally meaningful, extended beyond herself,

[1] Participants' names have been changed.

and was stable over time. The fact that Marta's purpose endured across adolescence and early emerging adulthood is noteworthy given the large shifts in identity and life circumstances that accompany these life stages (Arnett 2004). Despite moving away from home, working full-time while in school, and changing majors, Marta remained purposefully engaged in doing what she believed God had called her to do.

Familial Purpose

Just as religion can serve as both a source of purpose and a source of purposeful engagement, families too can represent personally meaningful aspirations and avenues for acting on highly valued aims. Serving one's family, providing for and loving one's offspring, and preserving one's family traditions represent varied manifestations of familial purpose. A familial purpose may also be evident among youth who harbor a strong desire to have a family in the future, and who in adolescence and emerging adulthood are already making school, dating, and career plans with a future family in mind. Purposeful engagement may be evident when an individual seeks to overturn ethnic stereotypes and does so in part by raising open-minded and free thinking children. Such an individual could pursue a life purpose, in part, by raising children in a particular way.

Empirical studies have determined that connectedness, is an important pre-requisite to discovering purpose. For example, studies report that individuals who feel close to others and to the social world are more likely to report having a purpose in life (Debats et al. 1995). At the same time, the lack of social relationships has been shown to result in purposelessness (Stillman et al. 2009). Similarly, meaninglessness is significantly associated with feelings of alienation and isolation (Debats et al. 1995), and interpersonal rejection has been shown to correlate with a loss in the perceived purposiveness of living (Sommer et al. 2012).

In spite of the significant association between feeling close to others and pursuing purpose, virtually no empirical studies have directly focused on what familial or relational purposes look like or how they function. Perhaps one reason familial purpose is under-studied is because most recent research on the construct has featured adolescent and emerging adult individuals, most of whom have not started a family yet. There are, of course, youth who are committed to providing for and serving their families of origin. In collectivistic cultures this is the norm, but in more autonomous, Western cultures it is less common. As such in Western cultures, it seems likely that familial purpose may be more prevalent among middle aged adults who have families of their own.

This possibility is supported by studies of parenting (Umberson and Gove 1989) and caregiving (Marks et al. 2002) that conclude that individuals who engage in these activities, typically associated with midlife report higher levels of purpose than non-parents and non-caregivers. However, while parenting and caregiving *may* be purposeful activities, they also may not be. Presumably, some caregivers and some parents, even attentive ones, provide the care they do out of a sense of obligation rather than a sense of purpose. When individuals fail to envision their relational roles in meaningful terms, they are not likely to report increased levels of purpose (McKnight and Kashdan 2009). In other words, being a member of a family it self that is purposeful but the way the individual orients to being a member of a family that determines whether the experience is purposeful.

Case Study of Familial Purpose The following example of familial and relational purpose emerged from a one-year longitudinal study with rural youth (Bronk et al., under review). This particular case study highlights the individual's devotion to supporting her family and nurturing that relationship. Perhaps not coincidentally, this individual is slightly older than the other interviewees and she has a child of her own.

Dana grew up physically and emotionally close to her parents, sister, and extended family. As a child and adolescent, her sister was her best friend and her parents and grandma served as trusted sources of wisdom and guidance. As an emerging adult, she became pregnant, and the love, help, and support she received from her family became even more important to her than before. At twenty-four years of age, when she was interviewed for the first time, she was an enthusiastic and doting mother of a two-year-old. Her gratitude and devotion to her family had grown to include her daughter. "My life revolves around [my daughter]." She explained that she hoped to instill in her daughter a deep love and sincere respect for family.

Wrapping up college, she planned to become an elementary school teacher. In explaining her choice of career paths, she highlighted the potential relationship she could build with her young students. As a teacher, she noted, "you're going to be shaping [children]," and she was eager to have a positive and lasting impact on her students' lives. She explained that, especially in the early elementary school years, teachers are like surrogate parents. Accordingly, effective teachers serve as "a shoulder to cry on" and an important source of "trust" and support.

Dana clearly places a high value on her personal relationships, and she appropriately organized her life, including her college and career plans, around them. In fact, when asked about her purpose, she insightfully said, "I would hope my purpose was to be a good mom, a good daughter, a good sister, and a good teacher and wife... but especially a good mom." It is interesting to note that all of her personally meaningful aims center on herself in relation to others. As such, she exemplifies relational, and especially familial, purpose.

Professional Purposes and Callings

In addition to finding purpose in families, many people find purpose in their paid word. Finding purpose here represents a "calling" or "vocation" (Damon 2008; Weiler and Schoonover 2001). Career or vocational purposes and callings are associated with greater happiness and well-being in life in general (Ryff and Singer 1998) and at work (Bonebright et al. 2000). Because of the clear relationship between purpose and happiness in the work place, programs designed to help adolescents (e.g., Dik et al. 2011; Kosine et al. 2008) and adults (e.g., Leider 1997) identify the things that matter most to them and connect their interests with possible career paths are fairly common. Purpose-centered approaches to career development typically aim to help individuals identify work that will be personally significant and at the same time allow them to make a useful contribution to the world beyond-themselves (Kosine et al. 2008). A more detailed discussion of empirically-based programs is included in Chap. 5 (Origins of and Supports for Purpose).

Beyond studies designed to support the development of purpose at work and connect individuals with careers that align with their aspirations, research on career-oriented purpose is limited, and more work in this area is needed. For example, studies to determine the kinds of professions most commonly associated with career or work purposes are warranted. It seems likely that purpose would be more prevalent among individuals pursuing helping professions—such as teaching, nursing, and social work—but this research has yet to be carried out, and it certainly is possible to derive purpose from other types of careers and jobs. Studies are also needed to explore how individuals pursuing purposeful careers approach their work. We know that they are less likely to show signs of workaholism and more likely to enjoy their jobs (Bonebright et al. 2000), but do they produce higher quality work products than individuals who lack purpose? Do they approach their jobs the same way as people without purpose? Do social supports or other resources in the workplace help them remain committed over time? Designing studies that address these questions and others would shed important light on the nature of professional purpose.

There are two plausible paths to pursuing a career-oriented purpose. Either, individuals discover a purpose and subsequently seek out a job or career that will allow them to make progress toward this aim, or individuals discover purposes through working. Though both paths seem likely, at present empirical evidence is only available to support the latter (Bronk 2012). For some individuals, work is not particularly meaningful at first, but over time it takes on greater meaning. For still others, work may represent not a purpose at all, but instead a form of purposeful engagement. A sample of pre-service teachers and nursing students reported selecting their professions because teaching youth and caring for patients represented important ways of helping others, and this was something that mattered deeply to them (Bronk et al., under review).

Case Study of Career Purpose It is not uncommon for young people to pursue purpose in their work (Bronk 2012). Neely is one such example. She was a nineteen-year-old college freshman from West Virginia when she was first interviewed. Attending college in New England, she was excited about pursuing a career in medicine. From the time she was in kindergarten, she had been involved in raising money to support cancer research. She sold daffodils and organized races to raise funds, and she created the first American Cancer Society Junior Board, so young people like her could get more deeply involved in the fight against cancer. Her volunteer efforts framed her childhood and adolescence and ultimately influenced her choice of careers.

Most broadly, Neeley's purpose revolved around helping people, but more specifically she aimed to do this by aiding people in getting the healthcare they needed. For Neely, her choice of careers was an outgrowth of her personal system of beliefs and values: "[Cancer fundraising helps] you see sort of your place in the world. You see how you're not just lost in the sea of things, how you actually can contribute and how you can somehow affect someone else's life in any regard and I think that that's necessary. We're not isolated people… That's what we really are supposed to be doing is helping someone else." The way Neely pursued this aim was through volunteering and preparing to work in the healthcare field.

> I'm very fascinated by the field of healthcare and by medicine, but I don't intend to be a practicing physician… I feel like my own skills and my own interests lie elsewhere, particularly on these social, political issues of healthcare, more managerial aspects than direct patient care… I'm actually doing an MD/MBA because… we still haven't figured out the best way to deliver healthcare in our country, and so I think I really want to focus on more of these broader social problems.

Neeley's career path provided a unique avenue for applying her particular skill set in service of a personally valued aim.

Artistic Purpose

Like many of the other types of purpose, artistic purposes have rarely been the focus of empirical research. One of the particular challenges in studying artistic purpose has to do with the self-oriented nature of the activity. People commonly create art because they enjoy it and through it they can express themselves. These self-oriented motivations are not sufficient for purpose, since a purpose represents a personally meaningful aim to contribute to the world *beyond-the-self*. That said, clearly some people pursue art, not only for what it can do for themselves, but also for what it can do for others, and studies designed to address questions of the nature, prevalence, and experience of artistic purpose are needed.

Case Study of Artistic Purpose Because of his ability to clearly articulate his motivations behind his artistic commitment, Paolo provides a particularly compelling example of artistic purpose. In three interviews with Paulo, he spoke at length about pursuing a life built around his love of jazz piano. His passion for music was clear. "[When you're playing] you're just expressing your emotions. Whatever you're thinking about, whatever you're feeling gets translated through your instrument and the process is really fun. It's really exciting." Self-oriented motivations for playing music are clearly evident here. However, his dedication was not only self-serving. "So I think I'd like to create music that [makes people think or experience something]. That gets people in touch with their emotions, and how they're really feeling… They might not be able to feel certain things quite so easily without being exposed to music." Paolo's dedication to jazz music is fueled in part by a desire to impact others, and accordingly, his commitment represents purpose.

Five years after his first interview, Paolo's, beyond-the-self motivations had further evolved. He talked about wanting to help broaden the audience for jazz music, and he hoped to leave his mark on the genre by combining his blossoming interest in electronic music with his deep knowledge of jazz piano.

Paolo began playing music when he was six, and his enthusiasm for music in general and jazz in particular grew over time. Though he had the opportunity to attend a highly competitive engineering school, he instead chose to attend a music college because at his core he considered himself a musician. "I identified with [jazz piano]. Oh, who's that guy? Oh, that's Paolo. He plays jazz piano. I didn't get oh, that's Paolo, he's good at math."

Artistic purposes vary widely, and Paolo provides an instructive example of only one manifestation of artistic purpose. His commitment was enduring, he sacrificed to advance his musical career, and he clearly sought to use his music not only for his own enjoyment, but also as a means of impacting others. Yet, because Paolo's commitment to music evolved into a career path, his purpose could be categorized not only as a form of artistic purpose, but also as a form of career purpose. This example underscores the challenge involved in clearly fitting purposes into only one category.

Civic and Political Purpose

Civic work, including political and community service activities, represents the last category of purpose. Interestingly, while many young people today are engaged in community service activities, relatively few are committed to political aims. A recent survey revealed that over 50 % of high school students volunteer in their communities at least monthly, and more than 25 % do so weekly (Youniss and Yates 1997), but political knowledge and political interest among youth today is remarkably low (Colby et al. 2007). Consequently, while service-oriented purposes are fairly prevalent, political purposes are particularly rare (Damon 2008).

As with research on other types of purpose, empirical studies of civic purpose are limited. Only a handful of studies directly address the topic. One of those studies determined that altruistic youth who engage in helping behaviors are not only more likely to report higher levels of well-being, (Benson et al. 2007), but are also more likely to report purpose than youth who are not altruistically engaged (Schwartz et al. 2009). Of course purposes do not need to be altruistic or prosocial in nature. For example, expanding the audience for jazz music is not necessarily a prosocial aim, but it does represent an intention to have an impact on the world beyond-the-self, and therefore, it is purposeful. However, while purpose need not be prosocial in nature, many purposes, especially civic purposes, are. Given the potential prosocial bent of a purpose, the finding that altruism and purpose are related is not particularly surprising. More surprising, however, is research that finds that high ability youth are more likely than typical youth to cite service-oriented purposes (Bronk et al. 2010). This study compared rates of purpose among students who attended a private school for the gifted with rates of purpose among students who attended a mainstream, public school. However, it seems likely that this finding underscores not a difference in intelligence, but in opportunity. The high ability school provided many more opportunities for engagement in community service activities and made clearer its expectations that all students would serve in some capacity.

Case Studies of Civic Purposes Civic purposes encompass both commitments to political engagement and community service; therefore, case studies of both political and service-oriented purposes are included here.

Mitch attended high school in Texas where he became fascinated by politics. Though he grew up in a politically conservative family, his parents were not particularly vocal about their political leanings. Mitch spent a good deal of time reflecting on his personal beliefs, and ultimately decided his personal values aligned more closely with conservative ideologies than liberal ones.

His interest in politics started with a high school civics teacher, who encouraged him to explore his beliefs and who challenged his ideas. Mitch became involved in different campus-based political groups, but it was not until he left for college that he became particularly active. Ironically, Mitch attended one of the most liberal universities in the country. He felt that his professors and friends had an unexamined liberal bias, and this bothered him, so he became more involved in the local College Republicans chapter. As his political involvement grew, he ran for and won a term as Chairman of the state-wide College Republicans. After college he worked on a Republican presidential campaign and for a conservative think tank. When we spoke with him last he was debating running for political office, but whether he decided to do that or not, he noted, "I'm making a difference and I'm fulfilling that, plus I'm involved in politics… [and] the work is fulfilling… I'm involved in at least things I think are greater than me and I am able to make a difference. And at this point I think I want to go into politics and I'm pretty sure I'll stay that route." Mitch's political aims offer him a means of impacting the broader world in a personally meaningful way.

Reid provides another illustrative example of civic purpose, but his commitment is to community service rather than political work. When Reid, a Canadian, was seven-years-old, his teacher told his class about the difficulty of obtaining clean drinking water in some third world countries. This lesson "really got through to" Reid, and he decided to learn more about how he could help. With the support of his parents and teacher, Reid discovered that if he raised enough money, he could help build a well that would provide clean water for an entire community. He tackled the challenge with a focus and persistence not commonly found among children his age. For over a year he did chores around the house, made speeches at local elementary schools, and participated in interviews with various media outlets, all in the interest of raising funds. After a year, he earned the money needed to build a well, and he contacted the relevant organization to make it happen. A well was built, but Reid did not stop there.

By the time Reid was interviewed, he twelve-years old. He had founded his own non-profit organization focused on supporting water projects around the world. Five years later, when he was interviewed again, his foundation had raised over a million dollars to build over 700 water projects around the world. "We're doing some good work," Reid noted in his final interview, "but there's still so much more work that needs to be done." When asked why he did all of this Reid explained that there are many significant problems, such as the lack of clean drinking water in parts of the world, and this was the one he felt equipped to tackle. He could have gone at it from a variety of perspectives, but his talent lay in fund raising. "No matter who you are, in whatever way you can [you can make a difference]. We've gotten help from people all across the world who, whether they just translate some stuff, help volunteer, and do work at the foundation are just doing their part to make the world a better place, in their own way. Because we're all not the same and we all need to contribute in different ways and I've really been impressed with how that has happened." Reid found a way of putting his talents to work in pursuit of a personally meaningful aim, and he made a significant difference.

It should be noted that with the exception of the familial purpose profile, the other profiles, including Mitch's and Reid's, feature youth purpose exemplars. Accordingly, these young people demonstrate exceptionally highly developed forms of purpose. Their commitments are intense, which makes them useful for illustrative purposes, but which can obscure the picture of more typical purpose. Individuals with somewhat weaker commitments to their personally meaningful aims may still demonstrate purpose. In fact, less pervasive forms of purpose are the norm. Chapter 8 (Youth Purpose Exemplars) includes a fuller discussion of the research conducted on this small sample and outlines some of strengths and weaknesses of studying exemplar samples.

With perhaps the exception of research on religious purpose, empirical studies of different types of purpose are clearly limited. It makes sense in a relatively new area of study, such as this, that examinations at a more granular level have not yet occurred. However, given that a clear definition of purpose exists and that the positive role of purpose in optimal human functioning has been established, now is the time. Examining various sources of inspiring purpose is critical to understanding how different kinds of purposes develop and how they can be effectively supported over time. Career purposes likely follow a distinct development a path and require different forms of encouragement than familial or religious purposes, for example. And civic and political purposes are likely associated with a different set of character strengths and positive psychological outcomes than say familial or religious purposes. Chapter 9 (Future Directions for Purpose Research) includes a more comprehensive and detailed discussion of the need for this line of inquiry.

In addition to gaining a clearer understanding of different types of purpose, it is also valuable to examine purpose among diverse groups of individuals. Youth from various ethnic, cultural, and geographic backgrounds are likely to vary in the way they commit to personally meaningful aims and in the kinds of aims to which they commit. The following chapter examines the experience of leading a life of purpose among diverse groups of individuals.

References

Allen, R. O., & Spilka, B. (1967). Committed and consensual religion, A specification of religion-prejudice relationships. *Journal for the Scientific Study of Religion, 6,* 191–206.

Allport, G. W., & Ross, J. M. (1967). Personal religious orientation and prejudice. *Journal of Personality and Social Psychology, 5,* 432–443.

Arnett, J. J. (2004). *Emerging adulthood: The winding road from late teens through the twenties.* New York: Oxford University Press.

Batson, C. D., & Ventis, W. L. (1982). *The religious experience: A social psychological perspective.* New York: Oxford University Press.

Baum, S. K., & Stewart, R. B. (1990). Sources of meaning through the lifespan. *Psychological Reports, 67,* 3–14.

Benson, P. L., Clary, E. G., & Scales, P. C. (2007). Altruism and health: Is there a link during adolescence? In S. G. Post (Ed.), *Altruism and health: Perspectives from empirical research.* (pp. 97–115). New York: Oxford University Press.

Bonebright, C. A., Clay, D. L., & Ankenmann, R. D. (2000). The relationship of workaholism with work-life conflict, life satisfaction, and purpose in life. *Journal of Counseling Psychology, 47,* 469–477.

Booth, A., Johnson, D. R., Branaman, A., & Sica, A. (1995). Belief and behavior: Does religion matter in today's marriages? *Journal of Marriage and Family, 57,* 661–671.

Bronk, K. C. (2005). Portraits of purpose: A grounded theory of the way purpose contributes to positive youth development. *Dissertation Abstracts International*, (UMI No. 3187267).

Bronk, K. C. (2011). Portraits of purpose: The role of purpose in identity formation. A special issue on Instructing for and Supporting Youth Purpose. *New Directions in Youth Development, 132,* 31–44.

Bronk, K. C. (2012). A grounded theory of youth purpose. *Journal of Adolescent Research, 27,* 78–109. doi:http://dx.doi.org/10.1177/0743558411412958.

Bronk, K. C., Finch, H. W., Kollman, J., & Youngs, A., (under review, Oct. 2012). Ecological and social support for rural youth purpose.

Bronk, K. C., Finch, W. H., & Talib, T. (2010). The prevalence of a purpose in life among high ability adolescents. *High Ability Studies, 21*(2), 133–145.

Byrd, K. R., Hagerman, A., & Isle, D. B. (2007). Intrinsic motivation and subjective well-being: The unique contribution of intrinsic religious motivation. *The International Journal for the Psychology of Religion, 17*(2), 141–156.

Chamberlain, K., & Zika, S. (1988). Religiosity, life meaning and well-being: Some relationships in a sample of women. *Journal for the Scientific Study of Religion, 27,* 411–420.

Clydesdale, T. T. (1997). Family behaviors among early U. S. baby boomers: Exploring the effects of religion and income change, 1965–1982. *Social Forces, 722,* 605–636.

Colby, A., Beaumont, E., Ehrlich, T., & Corngold, J. (2007). *Educating for democracy: Preparing undergraduates for responsible political engagement.* San Francisco: Jossey Bass.

Courtenay, B. C., Poon, L. W., Martin, P., Clayton, G. M., & Johnson, M. (1992). Religiosity and adaptation in the oldest-old. *International Journal of Aging and Human Development, 34*(1), 47–56.

Crandall, J. E., & Rasmussen, R. D. (1975). Purpose in life as related to specific values. *Journal of Clinical Psychology, 31,* 483–485.

Crumbaugh, J. C. (1968). Cross-validation of purpose in life test based on Frankl's concepts. *Journal of Individual Psychology, 24*(1), 74–81.

Crumbaugh, J. C., & Maholick, L. T. (1964). An experimental study in existentialism: The psychometric approach to Frankl's concept of noogenic neurosis. *Journal of Clinical Psychology, 20*(2), 200–207.

Crumbaugh, J. C., Raphael, S. M., & Shrader, R. R. (1970). Frankl's will to meaning in a religious order. *Journal of Clinical Psychology, 26,* 206–7.

Damon, W. (2008). *The path to purpose: Helping young people find their calling in life*. New York: Free Press.

Damon, W., Menon, J., & Bronk, K. C. (2003). The development of purpose during adolescence. *Applied Developmental Science, 7*(3), 119–128.

Davidson, J. D. (1972). Religious belief as an independent variable. *Journal for the Scientific Study of Religion, 11,* 65–75.

Debats, D. L., Drost, J., & Hansen, P. (1995). Experiences of meaning in life: A combined qualitative and quantitative approach. *British Journal of Psychology, 86,* 359–375.

DeVogler, K. L., & Ebersole, P. (1980). Categorization of college students' meaning in life. *Psychological Reports, 46,* 387–390.

DeVogler, K. L., & Ebersole, P. (1981). Adults' meaning in life. *Psychological Reports, 49,* 87–90.

DeVogler, K. L., & Ebersole, P. (1983). Young adolescents' meaning in life. *Psychological Reports, 52,* 427–431.

Dillon, M. (1999). The authority of the holy revisited: Habermas, religion, and emanciaptory possibilities. *Social Theory, 17*(3), 290–306.

Dik, B. J., Steger, M. F., Gibson, A., & Peisner, W. (2011). Make your work matter: Development and pilot evaluations of a purpose-centered career education intervention. *New Directions for Youth Development, 132,* 59–73.

Ebersole, P. (1998). Types and depth of written life meanings. In P. T. P. Wong (Ed.), *The human quest for meaning: A handbook of psychological research and applications* (2nd ed., pp. 179–191). New York: Routledge.

Emmons, R. A. (1999). *The psychology of ultimate concerns: Motivation and spirituality in personality*. New York: The Guilford Press.

Emmons, R. A. (2005). Striving for the sacred: Personal goals, life meaning, and religion. *Journal of Social Issues, 61,* 731–746.

Erikson, E. H. (1968). *Identity: youth and crisis*. New York: W. W. Norton.

Erikson, E. H. (1980). *Identity and the life cycle (paperback)*. New York: W.W. Norton.

Fletcher, S. K. (2004). Religion and life meaning: Differentiating between religious beliefs and religious community in constructing life meaning. *Journal of Aging Studies, 18,* 171–185.

Fowler, J. W. (1981). *Stages of faith: The psychology of human development and the quest for meaning*. New York: HarperCollins.

Francis, L. J. (2000). The relationship between Bible reading and purpose in life among 13–15 year olds. *Mental, Health, Religion, & Culture, 3,* 27–36.

Francis, L. J., & Burton, L. (1994). The influence of personal prayer on purpose in life among Catholic adolescents. *Journal of Beliefs and Values, 15,* 6–9.

Francis, L. J., & Evans, T. E. (1996). The relationship between personal prayer and purpose in life among churchgoing and non-churchgoing 12–15 year olds in the UK. *Religious Education, 91,* 9–21.

Francis, L. J., Jewell, A., & Robbins, M. (2010). The relationship between religious orientation, personality, and purpose in life among an older Methodist sample. *Mental Health, Religion & Culture, 13*(7–8), 777–791.

French, S., & Joseph, S. (1999). Religiosity and its association with happiness, purpose in life, and self-actualization. *Mental Health, Religion & Culture, 2*(2), 117–120.

George, L. K. (2000). Well-being and sense of self: What we know, what we need to know. In K. W. Shaie & J. Hendricks (Eds.), *The evolution of the aging self* (pp. 1–36). New York: Springer.

Koenig, H. G., Smiley, M., & Gonzales, J. A. P. (1988). *Religion, health, and aging: A review and theoretical integration*. Westport, CT: Greenwood Press.

Kosine, N. R., Steger, M. F., & Duncan, S. (2008). Purpose-centered career development: A strengths-based approach to finding meaning and purpose in careers. *Professional School Counseling, 12*(2), 133–136.

Leider, R. (1997). *The power of purpose: Creating meaning in your life and work*. San Francisco: Berrett-Koehler Publishers.

Mahoney, A., Pargament, K. I., Jewell, T., Swank, A. B., Scott, E., Emery, E., & Rye, M. (1999). Marriage and the spiritual realm: The role of proximal and distal religious constructs in marital functioning. *Journal of Family Psychology, 13,* 1–8.
Mariano, J. M., & Damon, W. (2008). The role spirituality and religious faith play in supporting purpose in adolescence. In R. M. Benson, R. W. Roeser & E. Phelps (Eds.), *Positive youth development and spirituality: From theory to research.* (pp. 210–230). West Conshoshocken, PA: Templeton Foundation Press.
Marks, N. F., Lambert, J. D., & Choi, H. (2002). Transitions to caregiving, gender, and psychological well-being: Prospective evidence from a U.S. national study. *Journal of Marriage and Family, 64,* 657–667.
Mc Knight, P. E., & Kashdan, T. (2009). Purpose in life as a system the creates and sustains health and well-being: An integrative, testable theory. *Review of General Psychology, 13*(3), 242–251.
Nozick, R. (1989). *The examined life: Philosophical meditations*. New York: Simon & Schuster.
Paloutzian, R. F. (1981). Purpose in life and value changes following conversion. *Journal of Personality and Social Psychology, 41*(6), 1153–1160.
Paloutzian, R. F., & Ellison, C. W. (1982). Loneliness, spiritual well-being, and quality of life. In L. A. Peplau & D. Perlman (Eds.), *Loneliness: A sourcebook, of current theory, research, and therapy*. New York: Wiley.
Pargament, K. I., & Park, C. L. (1995). Merely a defense? The variety of religious means and ends. *Journal of Social Issues, 51,* 13–32.
Prager, E. (1996). Exploring personal meaning in an age-differentiated Australian sample: Another look at the Sources of Meaning Profile (SOMP). *Journal of Aging Studies, 10*(2), 117–136.
Rathi, N., & Rastogi, R. (2007). Meaning in life and psychological well-being in pre-adolescents and adolescents. *Journal of the Indian Academy of Applied Psychology, 33*(1), 31–38.
Riley, M. W., Kahn, R. L., & Foner, A. (1994). *Age and structural lag: Society's failure to provide meaningful opportunities in work, family, and leisure*. New York: Wiley.
Robbins, M., & Francis, L. J. (2005). Purpose in life and prayer among Catholic and Protestant adolescents in Northern Ireland. *Journal of Research on Christian Education, 14*(1), 73–93.
Ryff, C., & Singer, B. (1998). The contours of positive human health. *Psychological Inquiry, 9*(1), 1–28.
Ryff, C. D., & Singer, B. (2008). Know thyself and become what you are: A eudaimonic approach to psychological well-being. *Journal of Happiness Studies, 9,* 13–39.
Schwartz, C. E., Keyl, P. M., Marcum, J. P., & Bode, R. (2009). Helping others shows differential benefits on health and well-being for male and female teens. *Journal of Happiness Studies, 10,* 431–448.
Soderstrom, D., & Wright, E. W. (1977). Religious orientation and meaning in life. *Journal of Clinical Psychology, 33,* 65–68.
Sommer, K. L., Baumeister, R. F., & Stillman, T. F. (2012). The construction of meaning from life events: Empirical studies of personal narratives. In P. T. P. Wong (Ed.), *The human quest for meaning: Theories, research, and applications*, (2nd ed., pp. 297–313). New York: Routledge.
Starck, P. L. (1999). Micro foundations of religion: A revised theory. *Sociological Theory, 17*(3), 264–289.
Steger, M. F., & Frazier, P. (2005). Meaning in life: One link in the chain from religiousness to well-being. *Journal of Counseling Psychology, 52*(4), 574–582.
Stillman, T. F., Baumeister, R. F., Lambert, N., Crescioni, A. W., DeWall, C. N., & Fincham, F. D. (2009). Alone and without purpose: Life loses meaning following social exclusion. *Journal of Experimental Social Psychology, 45,* 686–94.
Tillich, P. (1952). *The courage to be*. New Haven, CT: Yale University Press.
Tirri, K., & Quinn, B. (2010). Exploring the role of religion and spirituality in the development of purpose: Case studies of purposeful youth. *British Journal of Religious Education, 32*(3), 201–214.
Townsend, M., Kladder, V., Ayele, H., & Mulligan, T. (2002). Systematic review of clinical trials examining the effects of religion on health. *Southern Medical Journal, 95,* 1429–1434.

Umberson, D., & Gove, W. (1989). Parenthood and psychological well-being: Theory, measurement, and stage in the life course. *Journal of Family Issues, 10,* 440–462.

VanDyke, C. J., & Elias, M. J. (2007). How forgiveness, purpose, and religiosity are related to the mental health and well-being of youth. *Mental Health, Religion, & Culture, 10*(4), 395–415.

Weiler, N. W., & Schoonover, S. C. (2001). *Your soul at work: Five steps to a more fulfilling career and life*. Mahwah, NJ: Hidden Spring.

Wong, P. T. P., & Fry, P. S. (1998). Implicit theories of meaningful life and the development of the personal meaning profile. In P. T. P. Wong, & P. S. Fry (Eds.), *The human quest for meaning: A handbook of psychological research and clinical applications* (pp. 111–140). Mahwah, NJ: Lawrence Erlbaum Associates.

Youniss, J., & Yates, M. (1997). *Community service and social responsibility in youth.* Chicago: University of Chicago Press.

Chapter 7
The Experience of Purpose Among Diverse Groups

Affective Experience of Purpose

Based on research presented to this point, it is probably not surprising to learn that the experience of leading a life of purpose is generally a positive one. Individuals who have a purpose in life typically report positive emotions and positive emotional states (King et al. 2006). For instance, as discussed in greater detail in Chap. 3 (The Role of Purpose in Optimal Human Functioning), purpose is significantly associated with subjective well-being (Seligman 2002; Zika and Chamberlain 1987; Gillham et al. 2011), positive affect (King et al. 2006), hope (Bronk et al. 2010), and life satisfaction (Ho et al 2010; Bronk et al. 2009). While some forms of purpose are also associated with happiness (Soderstrom and Wright 1977), the construct is more commonly characterized by feeling as though one is leading the life he or she was meant to live (Bronk 2011). For instance, values such as salvation and virtues such as clean-living tend to be associated with the experience of purpose, while values such as pleasure, comfort, and excitement tend to be associated with the experience of purposelessness (Paloutzian 1981; Simmons 1980).

While the pursuit of purpose appears to be a positive experience, the discovery of purpose may not be. In some cases, searching for a purpose can be difficult and uncomfortable, especially when the search is carried out later in life (Bronk et al. 2009). In spite of the challenges associated with the search, however, Frankl (1959) believed that purpose could be discovered under any circumstances, including highly distressing and depressing ones.

As discussion in Chap. 3 (The Role of Purpose in Optimal Human Functioning), the relationship between purpose and positive affect is complex. Research that identifies the conditions under which purpose and positive affect are related needs to be conducted. Research designed to untangle the direction of the relationship, however has been conducted. To determine whether purpose *leads* to positive states or if being in a good mood *leads* to the development of purpose or meaning, researchers conducted a series of six studies (King et al 2006). The first study established that meaning in life was strongly, positively related to positive mood states and negatively related to negative mood states. The second study demonstrated that the strongest predictor of a day being experienced as meaningful was the amount of

K. C. Bronk, *Purpose in Life*, DOI 10.1007/978-94-007-7491-9_7,

positive affect experienced during that day. In other words, a sense that all is well appears to support the experience of leading a meaningful life. Subsequent studies determined that ratings of meaning in life increased when individuals were primed with positive mood concepts. Taken together, the evidence suggests that positive moods lead to the development of meaning, or at a minimum, positive moods predispose individuals to feeling as though their lives are meaningful. Put another way, it is likely that positive moods increase individuals' awareness of and sensitivity to the meaningfulness in any given situation (King et al. 2006).

As might be expected, further research similarly confirms that purposelessness is significantly associated with negative mood states. Empirical studies find, for example, that individuals who lack purpose often experience high levels of negative affect, including anxiety, boredom, and depression (Fahlman et al. 2009). Similarly, chronically bored individuals tend to lack purpose (Drob and Bernard 1988), and leaving meaningful life projects can lead to a feeling of being stuck in a chronic state of boredom (Bargdill 2000).

Interestingly, whereas positive moods tend to induce states of meaning, negative moods do not appear to induce states of purposelessness. Instead, empirical studies conclude that a lack of purpose *leads* to the experience of negative affect (Fahlman et al. 2009). To reach this conclusion, researchers first manipulated some participants' moods (happy or sad) as a control and other participants' perceptions of purpose (high or low). Results revealed that while changes in mood did not change participants' scores on boredom, changes in perceptions of purpose did.

Purposelessness has also been shown to be significantly associated with high levels of death anxiety and purposefulness to lower levels of death anxiety (Drolet 1990). This may be due, at least in part, to the fact that individuals with purpose feel as though they will live on through their accomplishments and contributions. Their personally meaningful work in the broader world allows them to achieve a sense of symbolic immortality. In this way, pursuing purpose serves as an important avenue for generativity, especially in midlife (Erikson 1959; McAdams and Logan 2004).

We can conclude from this discussion that the subjective experience of leading a life of purpose is generally positive while the subjective experience of leading a life devoid of purpose is generally negative. However, important exceptions exist. As discussed earlier in this book, caregiving (Marks et al. 2002) and parenting (Umberson and Gove 1989) represent two common kinds of purpose, especially prevalent in midlife, that are not associated with positive affect, but are associated with purpose. More research is needed to gain a clearer understanding of these and potentially other circumstances under which purpose is not associated with positive affect. Likewise, while a significant relationship between purposelessness and negative mood states clearly exists, there are likely to be exceptions here as well. Given that purpose is rare and that most people do not experience severe depression or intense boredom, it seems likely that there are at least some circumstances under which purposelessness does not predict negative states at all. Just as empirical studies of purpose and negative affect are called for, so too are additional studies of purposelessness and positive or at least neutral affect needed. Gaining a fuller understanding of the circumstances under which these relationships exist would further illuminate our understanding of the complexities and limitations of the purpose construct.

Mechanism Responsible for the Affective Experience of Purpose In spite of these exceptions, the existing research suggests that for most people, most of the time, the experience of leading a life of purpose is a positive one, but it is not immediately clear why this is the case. It is also not evident if a particular component of purpose is responsible for these positive associations, and if this is the case, which component it is.

Theoretical and empirical research suggests there may be several potential mechanisms behind the relationship between positive emotions and purpose. The first has to do with the goal-oriented aspect of purpose. As discussed in greater detail in Chap. 1 (Introduction and Definition), a purpose in life represents a long-term, personally meaningful goal of sorts, and goal pursuit is strongly associated with positive feelings. For instance, a month-long study in which undergraduates were asked to keep diaries of goal attainment, goal importance, and subjective well-being in daily situations revealed that goal attainment and goal importance were significantly related to positive emotions (Emmons and Diener 1986). Since individuals with purpose by definition hold a goal of great personal importance and because they are necessarily engaged in working toward its attainment, it seems logical to expect that this aspect of the construct plays a key role in the positive affective experience of leading a life of purpose.

Second, inherent in goal pursuit is a strong sense of intrinsic motivation. Individuals who pursue goals tend to be highly motivated, and individuals with purpose are no exception. In fact, individuals with purpose report feeling strongly motivated—compelled even—to pursue their personally meaningful aims (Bronk 2005, 2012). Not surprisingly, research finds that highly motivated individuals report higher purpose scores (Crumbaugh et al. 1970), and individuals who are highly motivated to work toward a goal, such as a purpose, tend to feel better about their lives. For instance, research finds that individuals who are involved in goal-oriented activities such as personal projects (Little 1983) that are meaningful, manageable, and supported by others exhibit fewer signs of depression and more signs of well-being (Little 1989; Salmela-Aro and Nurmi 1997). This model suggests that the motivation inherent in pursuing a life of purpose may also be at least partially responsible for the relationship between purpose and positive feelings.

The third facet of the purpose construct likely to contribute to positive feelings is the beyond-the-self dimension. Individuals who aspire to a purpose in life do so at least in part out of a desire to contribute to matters larger than the self, and empirical research suggests that this commitment may be at least party responsible for the positive experience of leading a life of purpose. A recent study examined adolescent characteristics based on the type of long-term aims they held (Bronk and Finch 2010). One hundred and forty-four adolescent participants were categorized into one of three groups based on the type of long-term aim to which they aspired, including self-oriented long-term aims, beyond-the-self long-term aims, and aims that were both self-oriented and beyond-the-self in nature. Youth with goals that included a beyond-the-self component scored significantly higher on life satisfaction than youth who reported long-term aims that were exclusively self-oriented.

Along these same lines, a study engaged undergraduates in a diary writing task in which participants wrote about their activities and their corresponding emotions for a three-week period (Steger et al. 2007). Responses were categorized into two groups of activities: eudaimonic activities, which were primarily other-focused, and hedonic activities, which were primarily self-focused. Results revealed that engagement in eudaimonic activities, as compared to hedonic ones, correlated with higher scores of life meaning, positive affect, and life-satisfaction.

Lastly, a retrospective study examined beyond-the-self intentions among a sample of men who served in World War II (Mariano and Vaillant 2012). The researchers analyzed historical documents, including interviews conducted with these individuals when they were emerging adults. A textual analysis of those documents revealed that the men who expressed beyond-the-self concerns, as compared to the men who did not, were more likely to report having more positive experiences.

Social Experience of Purpose

Just as the affective experience of leading a life of purpose appears to be positive, so too does the social experience. In particular, close relationships appear to coincide with purposefulness (Padelford 1974; Reker 1977). Individuals tend to connect personally meaningful experiences to helping and caring interactions with a variety of people, including family, friends, and strangers (Debats et al. 1995). What is more, married individuals report higher purpose scores than single individuals (Zeitchik 2000), and altruistic adolescent males and females report more positive social relations and higher purpose scores than less altruistic individuals (Schwartz et al. 2009).

At the same time, social isolation is significantly associated with the experience of purposelessness. In particular, several studies have concluded that purposelessness predicts social anomie and alienation (Debats et al. 1995; Morojele and Brooks 2004; Ross and Mirowsky 2009). One such study asked participants to describe meaningless situations and the pictures participants painted consistently featured instances of separation and isolation from the broader social world (Debats et al. 1995). Another team of researchers concluded that purpose scores dropped following experiences of social exclusion (Stillman et al 2009).

One situation in which individuals often experience a sense of alienation or isolation is when they find themselves surrounded by people from different ethnic backgrounds. Demographic heterogeneity can make people feel threatened and ill at ease (Alesina and La Ferrara 2002). The constrict theory (Putnam 2007) suggests that people in ethnically diverse settings often choose to "hunker down" and form fewer social connections overall, including with people perceived to be like themselves and with people perceived to be different from themselves. Given the clear relationship between purpose and social connectedness, researchers wanted to see if individuals with purpose would feel isolated when surrounded by people from different ethnic backgrounds or if the experience would diminish their sense of purpose.

Researchers designed an innovative study to assess these possibilities. The study aimed to determine if having purpose influenced the way people felt in situations where they were surrounded by ethnically diverse others (Burrow 2012). Participants completed surveys of purpose and emotions and then boarded public transportation trains and traveled around a large metropolitan city in the United States. Unbeknownst to the participants, confederates rode the trains along with them and recorded the ethnic backgrounds of the other passengers. Once at their destination, participants again completed surveys of, among other things, purpose emotions. Whereas individuals without purpose tended to report higher levels of negative affect when they were on particularly diverse trains, individuals with purpose did not. In fact, their baseline scores of negative affect were lower than the baseline scores of individuals without purpose, and their negative affect scores did not significantly increase after being exposed to highly diverse environments. In other words, individuals with a purpose in life experienced less negative emotion initially and less negative emotion following the experience of being surrounded by people from different ethnic backgrounds. This finding suggests that pursuing a purpose in life may buffer individuals from potentially disorienting situations in which people from different ethnic backgrounds surround them.

To extend their findings regarding the social experience of purpose, researchers repeated the study, but this time they induced a state of purposefulness among the experimental group by asking these participants to write about their personally meaningful aspirations (Burrow 2012). Members of the control group wrote about their favorite movies. Then participants from both the experimental and control groups rode the trains while anonymous confederates recorded the ethnic backgrounds of the other passengers. After the train ride, participants again completed surveys of purpose and emotions. Individuals who had been primed to feel purposeful reported lower levels of negative affect after riding on trains with both low and high levels of diversity. Accordingly, it is evident that inducing a state of purpose protected these participants from the potentially negative feelings that often accompany social contexts characterized by high ethnic diversity.

Interestingly, this does not seem to be merely a Western phenomenon. A study of Chinese students studying abroad in Australia similarly concluded that individuals who reported high levels of meaning in life experienced lower rates of acculturative stress as compared to individuals who reported low meaning levels (Pan et al. 2008).

Self-Focused Experience of Purpose

In addition to feeling more comfortable in ethnically diverse contexts, individuals with a clear sense of purpose in life also tend to feel more comfortable with themselves. They tend to hold more positive self-concepts (Reker 1977) and experience higher levels of self-confidence (Crumbaugh and Maholick 1969; Crumbaugh et al. 1970), self-control (Crumbaugh and Maholick 1969), self-acceptance (Crumbaugh and Maholick 1969), and self-esteem (Bigler et al. 2001; Paloutzian and Ellison 1982; Schlesinger et al. 1990; Scannell et al. 2002) than individuals without purpose. Individuals with purpose also report closer alignment between the way they see themselves and they way they view their ideal selves (Reker 1977).

Experiences of meaningfulness are also associated with a greater sense of self-integration, while experiences of meaninglessness tend to be associated with a sense of personal disintegration (Debats et al. 1995). To reach this conclusion, researchers asked participants to describe instances in which their lives felt particularly meaningful and particularly meaningless. In describing times when their lives felt meaningless, participants pointed to experiences where they felt their potential was blocked and their disabilities held them back, and in describing times when their lives felt meaningful, participants discussed instances where they experienced a strong sense of self-unity.

In addition to experiencing positive moods, positive relations, and a sense of self-integration, individuals with purpose are also more likely to effectively manage stress than individuals without purpose. Individuals with purpose tend to be exposed to more stressors than individuals without purpose, but for a variety of reasons explained more fully in Chap. 3 (The Role of Purpose in Optimal Human Functioning), they tend to be better equipped to manage that stress.

One reason individuals with purpose are less likely to experience the negative effects of stress has to do with the increased sense of control they experience. Compared to individuals without purpose, purposeful individuals tend to view themselves as in control of their environment and less at the mercy of luck or chance (Reker 1977; Yarnell 1971). Leading a life of purpose has been associated with an internal locus of control (Pizzolato et al. 2011). An empirical study of meaning among South Africans found that individuals from lower socioeconomic backgrounds were more likely than wealthier individuals to report that their country's sociopolitical situation was meaningless (Morojele and Brooks 2004). It seems likely that individuals from more challenging backgrounds are feel helpless to change the way their country is governed, and; therefore, more likely to report feeling as though the whole situation is meaningless. Viewed from this perspective, this finding lends additional support to the connection between purpose and locus of control.

The Experience of Searching for Purpose

The discussion to this point has focused exclusively on individuals who have committed to a purpose in life. It has excluded the experience of searching for purpose. As it turns out, the latter experience can be quite different. Chapter 3 (The Role of Purpose in Optimal Human Functioning) includes a more complete discussion of the experience of searching for purpose, but in short, the search is associated with life satisfaction when it is carried out in adolescence and emerging adulthood, but not when it is carried out in midlife (Bronk et al. 2009).

Once individuals discover a purpose for their lives, we might expect them to spend less time searching for one. As outlined in Chap. 2 (Measuring Purpose), this is what Crumbaugh (1977) expected to find when he created the Seeking of Noetic Goals test (SONG; Crumbaugh 1977), which measures the motivation to find purpose, to complement his Purpose in Life test (PIL; Crumbaugh and Maholick 1964, 1969), which measures the degree to which individuals have already discovered a purpose. As he expected, an inverse relationship emerged among a sample of more typical individuals, but not among a sample of individuals being treated for psychological problems (Crumbaugh 1977). Crumbaugh interpreted this result as a sign that his newly created SONG measure adequately distinguished between psychologically healthy and unhealthy samples. Other researchers, however, have found that the search for purpose and the commitment to purpose are not necessarily incompatible (Bronk et al. 2009; Steger et al. 2007). In fact, some have argued that the two constructs may actually function independently, whereby individuals who have purpose in their lives continue to seek additional sources of meaning as the nature of their engagement changes (Steger et al. 2008a) or as additional ways of making progress toward their purposes emerge (Bronk 2012). In this latter view, the experience of having a purpose in life evolves over time. The way individuals pursue purpose in adolescence may not be the same way they do in adulthood, even though they may still aspire to the same far-horizon aim.

It is still unclear, however, why certain measures of purpose and the motivation to find purpose demonstrate an inverse relationship between the two constructs while other measures reveal that the constructs function independently. An explanation for this discrepancy may be found by looking more closely at the actual questions posed by the different measures. The searching questions in the Meaning in Life Questionnaire (MLQ; Steger et al. 2006) and the Revised Youth Purpose Survey (RYPS: Bundick et al. 2006), both of which find that the commitment to and the search for purpose function independently, include questions that specifically and directly assess the search for meaning and purpose in life (e.g., MLQ: "I am looking for something that makes my life feel meaningful" and RYPS: "I am always looking to find my life's purpose"). A high score on either of these questions points specifically to a strong motivation to search for meaning or purpose in life. The searching questions in the SONG (Crumbaugh 1977), which find an inverse relationship between a commitment to and a continued search for purpose, are much more general in nature (e.g., SONG; "I am restless" and "I feel that some element which I cannot quite define is missing from my life"). A high score on the SONG, therefore, implies a more generalized sense of unrest, disquiet, or searching rather than a specific search for purpose or meaning. Because the former two measures specifically probe the search for purpose and meaning, while the latter probes a more generalized sense of exploration, it is not surprising to find that they come to different conclusions. The fact that a vague sense of dissatisfaction or restlessness is inversely related to the presence of purpose is bolstered by other studies that find that purpose and anxiety, which similarly can be experienced as a sense of disquiet and restlessness, are also significantly inversely related (Bigler et al. 2001).

Some have also argued that the experience of searching for purpose varies based on one's cultural background (Steger et al. 2008b). Researchers have concluded that the presence of purpose and meaning are closely aligned with the way individuals view themselves in relation to the broader society (Baumeister 1991; Bronk 2011; Damon 2008; Erikson 1959, 1968). Individualistic cultures emphasize the self as an independent agent, whereas collectivistic cultures emphasize the inter-dependence among members (Heine et al. 2001). People from individualistic cultures are motivated to employ strategies that help support and sustain positive feelings about themselves (e.g., Heine et al. 1999; Oishi and Diener 2003), and as such, they are likely to place a higher value on committing to a purpose, which is associated with more positive feelings, than on the search for purpose, which is only associated with positive feelings at certain stages in the lifespan (Bronk et al. 2009). People from collectivistic cultures place a higher value on effort and striving for self-improvement (e.g., Heine et al. 1999; Oishi and Diener 2003). This process is more akin to the search for purpose, and as such, individuals from these cultures may feel more comfortable searching for a purpose than they do committing to one. Evidence in support of this theory exists. For example, Americans (independent culture) report higher levels of meaning in life than Japanese (collectivistic culture), and Japanese report higher levels of searching for meaning than Americans (Steger et al. 2008b). Americans also score higher on well-being, of which purpose is a prominent component, than Koreans (Ryff 1995). While additional cross-cultural studies are needed that examine both the process of searching for and committing to purpose among a wider range of cultures, it is evident that individuals from independent and collectivistic cultures experience the search for purpose and the presence of purpose differently.

Experience and Prevalence of Purpose Among Different Groups of People

Our discussion thus far has sought to provide a clearer picture of what leading a life of purpose is like for typical individuals, but this focus on "typical individuals" obscures interesting and important differences with regards to the nature and prevalence of purpose among diverse groups of individuals. Research on purpose has just begun to investigate the prevalence and forms of purpose among individuals from different backgrounds.

Across the lifespan, rates of purpose among Western individuals have been fairly well established (and are discussed in greater detail in Chap. 4, The Development of Purpose). In short, purpose generally emerges during adolescence and emerging adulthood (Bronk et al. 2009; Damon 2008; Reker 1977). From its peak in emerging adulthood, it tends to drop slightly among midlife adults and more significantly among later adults as opportunities for purposeful engagement disappear (Meier and Edwards 1974; Pearson and Sheffield 1974; Ryff 1995; Ryff and Singer 2008). This trend in the prevalence of purpose supports Frankl's (1959) belief that purposes are not given but discovered, and discovering a purpose for one's life takes time and requires opportunities for active engagement in potentially purposeful pursuits (Bronk 2012). Behind this larger trend, however, is a more detailed picture of who has purpose and of how these different groups of individuals experience a life of purpose. Factors such as country of origin, ethnic minority status, community type, and student status make a difference in the likelihood that an individual will discover and commit to a meaningful purpose in life.

Purpose Among Non-Western Individuals As noted previously, the vast majority of research on purpose has been carried out with Western participants (Jonsen et al 2010). However, a handful of cultural and cross-cultural studies have examined rates of purpose among individuals from different countries. For example, the Purpose in Life test was translated into Chinese and administered to a sample of Chinese adolescents (Shek et al. 1987). Results reveal that rates of purpose are comparatively lower among Chinese adolescents than among Western youth. The authors surmise that these results may be attributable to an authoritarian personality profile, which features a generally pessimistic attitude, common in the Chinese culture (Meade 1970; Meade and Barnard 1973). They may also be the result of the higher external locus of control typical among many Chinese (Yang 1981).

As discussed earlier in this chapter, lower rates of purpose have also been found among individuals from other Asian cultures. Koreans (Ryff 1995) report lower rates of well-being, of which purpose is a significant component, and Japanese report lower rates of purpose, but higher rates of searching for purpose than Americans (Steger et al. 2008b).

Social Inequality and Purpose In addition to focusing primarily on rates of purpose among Western individuals, research has also most commonly focused on purpose among students, a relatively privileged group. Few studies have explored purpose among individuals who experience social inequality. Frankl (1959) proposed that experiencing challenges in life, potentially associated with social inequality, did not preclude one from finding a purpose in life. In fact, he highlighted the life sustaining power of his own purpose during his incarceration in a Nazi concentration camp. Adversity, he argued, may actually contribute to a deepened sense of purpose in life.

Ryff et al. (2003) were eager to explore the experience of purpose based on social inequality, as measured by ethnic minority status, educational attainment, and perceived discrimination. Results suggest that ethnic minority status alone does not predict higher purpose scores, but that when education is added to the equation, it does. Highly educated African–Americans report higher purpose scores than highly educated Caucasians (Ryff et al. 2003). Educational attainment may serve as an important signal of status attainment, especially among ethnic minorities, and it can lead to increased opportunities in the workplace that may facilitate the pursuit of purpose, especially career-oriented and familial-support purposes. It has been proposed that educational attainment may equip ethnic minorities with cognitive and emotional skills that help them deal with racism (Ryff et al. 2003).

Purpose Among Ethnic Minorities Other studies suggest ethnic identity status is another important factor to consider with regards to purpose. A study of over 12,000 adolescents found that ethnic identity formation represented an important factor in whether or not ethnic minority individuals committed to a purpose (Martinez and Dukes 1997). This study found that ethnic minority youth with more advanced ethnic identity formation scores also reported higher purpose scores. For members of the majority status, ethnic identity is often taken for granted. It is rarely considered by these youth, and as such it rarely serves as a potential barrier to the development of purpose. Consequently, this study concluded that rates of purpose were higher among the majority Caucasian youth than among any of the ethnic minority youth, but among ethnic minority youth, purpose scores were higher for those youth who had made more progress in their ethnic identity development. While this correlation study does not allow for conclusions regarding the causal relationship between purpose and ethnic identity development, it does underscore the important relationship between purpose development and identity formation elaborated upon in Chap. 4 (The Development of Purpose).

We can conclude from this discussion that, consistent with Frankl's (1959) belief, challenges associated with status inequality and ethnic minority status do not inhibit the development of purpose, at least not when individuals are able to frame these challenges as personally meaningful. Frankl was careful to point out that "it is not suffering per se but suffering without meaning that is devastating to the individual" (p. 288). In other words, challenges, when viewed from the perspective of personal meaningfulness, do not necessarily curtail, and may even spur, the development of purpose.

While it appears to be the case that ethnic minority status does not preclude purpose, we still do not know much about the prevalence or nature of purpose among individuals from different ethnic and cultural backgrounds. This gap in the research highlights a significant oversight. A fuller discussion of the more specific types of studies needed and the significance of these studies is included in Chap. 9 (Future Directions for Purpose Research).

Purpose Among Individuals from Different Types of Communities Just as growing up in different cultures infuences the experience of purpose, so too does growing up in different sub-cultures and different kinds of communities. A series of studies examined the prevalence of purpose among youth from urban, suburban, and rural hometowns in the United States. Interestingly, urban and suburban youth report roughly the same rates of purpose and developed purposes at nearly the same time. Among early adolescents from urban and suburban hometowns, approximately 15 % reported a purpose in life, among late adolescents approximately a quarter do, and among emerging adults slightly more than a third do (Damon 2008). However, as is discussed in greater detail in Chap. 5 (Origins-of and Supports for Purpose), rates of purpose are significantly higher among late adolescent rural youth (Bronk et al. under review). A recent study revealed that 40 % of these young people (as compared to 25 % of youth from urban and suburban backgrounds) report having a clear in life purpose; and one reason likely has to do with the increased level of social support rural youth receive.

Purpose Among Incarcerated Individuals Researchers have also examined the prevalence of purpose among incarcerated individuals. Perhaps not surprisingly, individuals in jail report lower rates of purpose than individuals who are not in jail, and repeat offenders report lower rates of purpose than first-time offenders (Black and Gregson 1973; Reker 1977). While we do not know for sure why incarcerated individuals report lower purpose scores, we do know that aspects of the experience of the being in jail are associated with lower purpose scores. For example, given the monotonous experience of being in jail, it seems likely that boredom, which is associated with low purpose scores, may play a role. Also responsible for this finding may be the inmate's locus of control. Individuals in jail have little control over their lives and presumably experience an external locus of control, which has been associated with lower purpose scores (Pizzolato et al. 2011).

Purpose Among Students Lastly, having purpose also appears to play a special role in the lives of students. Given that the development of purpose typically corresponds with the development of identity associated with adolescence and emerging adulthood (Damon 2008; Erikson 1959, 1968), a growing body of research has investigated the role of purpose among secondary and college aged students. Empirical studies conclude that youth of school age who are in school report higher levels of purpose than youth who have dropped-out (Maton 1990). Of course, it is impossible to know if their low levels of purpose contributed to an over-riding sense of meaningless, thereby spurring them to drop out of school, or if they dropped out of school and subsequently realized that they were unlikely to be able to attain their aspirations without an education. It may also be the case that a third factor, such as homelessness, inhibits the pursuit of academic achievement and purpose. Regardless, of the direction of causality, the significant association between being in school and the pursuit of purpose is noteworthy.

Similar studies reveal that students who have purposeful work goals often report that their schoolwork is more meaningful (Yeagar and Bundick 2009). This finding suggests that a lack of purpose may lead individuals to drop out of school, rather than the other way around. Students who do not find meaning in the work they are doing are less likely to persevere at that work, and may be more likely—in extreme cases—to drop out of school. This finding also supports the academic stress theory put forth by Damon (2008, 2011) and discussed in Chap. 3 (The Role of Purpose in Optimal Human Functioning): work that is experienced as meaningful is not likely to be perceived as stressful, even when it may appear to others to be stress inducing. Lending additional support to this latter claim is the finding that higher purpose scores are associated with better grades among secondary education students (Benson 2008; Pizzolato et al. 2011)

Interestingly, however, purpose does not appear to be more common among high ability individuals than among more typical students. Research designed to assess the forms and prevalence of purpose among a sample of high ability adolescent and emerging adult students reveals that these youth commit to purposes at roughly the same time and rate as more typical individuals (Bronk et al. 2010). Other studies have similarly concluded that IQ scores do not predict purpose (Crumbaugh and

Maholick 1969; Yarnell 1971), except among inmates (Reker 1977). The relationship between grade point average and purpose among inmates may be attributable to the particularly large range in IQ scores evident among this sample (range 72–122) and suggests that additional research with samples that vary significantly in terms of intelligence is needed.

In sum additional research into the experience of purpose among typical individuals and diverse groups of individuals is needed. In particular, studies should examine the nature, prevalence, forms, and development of purpose among individuals from different ethnic and cultural backgrounds. Research on socioeconomic differences associated with the pursuit of purpose would also help illuminate our understanding of the construct.

While this chapter has shed light on the experience of purpose among different groups of individuals, it has largely ignored one important group. Youth who possess a particularly highly developed form of purpose are rarely included in empirical studies of the construct, and this represents a significant oversight. Youth purpose exemplars provide a useful picture of complete or nearly complete development of purpose. The following chapter includes an overview of what the exemplar methodology is, a discussion of its relevance to the study of youth purpose, and a synthesis of some of the significant findings that have emerged from a longitudinal study of youth purpose exemplars.

References

Alesina, A., & La Ferrara, E. (2002). Who trusts others? *Journal of Public Economics, 85*(2), 207–234.

Bargdill, R. (2000). The study of life boredom. *Journal of Phenomenological Psychology, 31*(2), 188–219.

Baumeister, R. (1991). *Meanings of life*. New York: Guilford Press.

Benson, P. L. (2008). *Sparks: How parents can help ignite the hidden strengths of teenagers*. San Francisco: Jossey Bass.

Bigler, M., Neimeyer, G. J., & Brown, E. (2001). The divided self revisited: Effects of self–concept clarity and self–concept differentiation on psychological adjustment. *Journal of Social and Clinical Psychology, 20*(3), 396–415.

Black, W. A. M., & Gregson, R. A. M. (1973). Time perspectives, purpose in life, extroversion, and neuroticism in New Zealand prisoners. *British Journal of Social and Clinical Psychology, 12*(1), 50–60.

Bronk, K. C. (2005). Portraits of purpose: A grounded theory of the way purpose contributes to positive youth development. *Dissertation Abstracts International*, (UMI No. 3187267).

Bronk, K. C. (2011). Portraits of purpose: The role of purpose in identity formation. *New directions for youth development, 132,* 31–44.

Bronk, K. C. (2012). A grounded theory of youth purpose. *Journal of Adolescent Research, 27*(1), 78–109. (http://dx.doi.org/10.1177/0743558411412958).

Bronk, K. C., & Finch, W. H. (2010). Adolescent characteristics by type of long–term aim in life. *Applied Developmental Science, 14*(1), 35–44.

Bronk, K. C., Hill, P. L., Lapsley, D. K., Talib, T., & Finch, W. H. (2009). Purpose, hope, and life satisfaction in three age groups. *Journal of Positive Psychology, 4*(6), 500–510.

Bronk, K. C., Finch, W. H., & Talib, T. (2010). The prevalence of a purpose in life among high ability adolescents. *High Ability Studies, 21*(2), 133–145.

Bronk, K. C., Finch, W. H., Kollman, J., & Youngs, A. (under review, 2012, December). Purpose in life among rural youth and the role of ecological and social support.

Bundick, M., Andrews, M., Jones, A., Mariano, J. M., Bronk, K. C., & Damon, W. (2006). *Revised youth purpose survey*. Unpublished instrument, Stanford Center on Adolescence, Stanford, CA.

Burrow, A. L. (2012). *Derailed by diversity?: The role of purpose in negotiating ethnically diverse contexts*. Paper symposium at the biennial meeting of the Society for Research on Adolescence, Vancouver, British Columbia.

Crumbaugh, J. C. (1977). The seeking of noetic goals test (SONG): A complimentary scale to the purpose in life test (PIL). *Journal of Clinical Psychology, 33*(3), 900–907.

Crumbaugh, J. C., & Maholick, L. T. (1964). An experimental study in existentialism: The psychometic approach to Frankl's concept of noogenic neurosis. *Journal of Clinical Psychology, 20,* 200–207.

Crumbaugh, J. C., & Maholick, L. T. (1969). *Manual for instructions for the purpose in life test*. Munster: Psychometric Affiliates.

Crumbaugh, J. C., Raphael, S. M., & Shrader, R. R. (1970). Frankl's will to meaning in a religious order. *Journal of Clinical Psychology, 26,* 206–7.

Damon, W. (2008). *The path to purpose: Helping our children find their calling in life*. San Francisco: Jossey Bass.

Damon, W. (2011, November 18). Getting off the treadmill: Finding purpose, by Terry Lobdell. *Palo Alto Daily News*, 37–48.

Debats, D. L., Drost, J., & Hansen, P. (1995). Experiences of meaning in life: A combined qualitative and quantitative approach. *British Journal of Psychology, 86,* 359–375.

Drob, S., & Bernard, H. (1988). The bored patient: A developmental existential perspective. *The Psychotherapy Patient, 3,* 63–73.

Drolet, J. (1990). Transcending death during early adulthood: Symbolic immortality, death anxiety, and purpose in life. *Journal of Clinical Psychology, 46*(2), 148–160.

Emmons, R. A., & Diener, E. (1986). A goal–affect analysis of situational choice and avoidance. *Journal of Research in Personality, 20,* 309–326.

Erikson, E. H. (1959). *Identity and the life cycle*. New York: W.W. Norton & Company Inc.

Erikson, E. H. (1968). *Identity: Youth and crisis*. New York: W.W. Norton & Company Inc.

Fahlman, S. A., Merce, K. B., Gaskovski, P., Eastwood, A. E., & Eastwood, J. D. (2009). Does a lack of life meaning cause boredom? Results from psychometric, longitudinal and experimental analyses. *Journal of Social and Clinical Psychology, 28*(3), 307–340.

Frankl, V. E. (1959). *Man's search for meaning: An introduction to logotherapy*. Boston: Beacon.

Gillham, J., Adams–Deutsch, Z., Werner, J., Reivich, K., Coulter–Heindl, V., Linkins, M., Winder, B., Peterson, C., Park, N., Abenavoli, R., Contero, A., & Seligman, M. E. P. (2011). Character strengths predict subjective well–being during adolescence. *Journal of Positive Psychology, 6*(1), 31–44. doi: 10.1080/17439760.2010.536773..

Heine, S. J., Kitayama, S., & Lehman, D. R. (2001). Cultural differences in self–evaluation: Japanese readily accept negative self–relevant information. *Journal of Cross–Cultural Psychology, 32,* 434–443.

Heine, S. J., Lehman, D. R., Markus, H. R., & Kitayama, s. (1999). Is there a universal need for positive self-regard? *Psychological Review, 106*(4) 766–794.

Ho, M. Y., Cheung, F. M., & Cheug, S. F. (2010). The role of meaning in life and optimism in promoting well–being. *Personality and individual differences, 48*(5), 658–663.

Jonsen, E., Fagerstrom, L., Lundman, B., Nygren, B., Vahakangas, M., & Strandberg, G. (2010). Psychometric properties of the Swedish version of the purpose in life scale. *Scandinavian Journal of Caring Science, 24,* 41–48.

King, L. A., Hicks, J. A., Krull, J. L., & Del Graiso, A. K. (2006). Positive affect and the experience of meaning in life. *Journal of Personality and Social Psychology, 90*(1), 179–196.

Little, B. R. (1983). Personal projects: A rationale and method for investigation. *Environment and Behavior, 15,* 273–309.
Little, B. R. (1989). Personal projects analysis: Trivial pursuits, magnificent obsessions, and the search for coherence. In D. M. Buss, & N. Cantor (Eds.), *Personality psychology: Recent trends and emerging directions* (pp. 15–31). New York: Springer.
Mariano, J. M., & Valliant, G. E. (2012). Youth purpose among the "Greatest Generation". *Journal of Positive Psychology*. doi:10.1080/17439760.2012.686624
Marks, N. F., Lambert, J. D., & Choi, H. (2002). Transitions to caregiving, gender, and psychological well–being: A prospective U.S. national study. *Journal of Marriage and Family, 64,* 657–67.
Martinez, R. O., & Dukes, R. L. (1997). The effects of ethnic identity, ethnicity, and gender on adolescent well–being. *Journal of Youth and Adolescence, 26*(5), 503–516.
Maton, K. I. (1990). Meaningful involvement in activity and well–being: Studies of older adolescents and at risk urban teen-agers. *American Journal of Community Psychology, 18*(2), 297–320.
McAdams, D. P., & Logan, R. L. (2004). What is generativity? In E. de St. Aubin. In D. P. McAdams, & T. C. Kim (Eds.), *The generative society* (pp. 15–31). Washington, DC: American Psychological Association.
Meade, R. D. (1970). Leadership studies of Chinese and Chinese–Americans. *Journal of Cross–Cultural Psychology, 1,* 325–332.
Meade, R. D., & Barnard, W. A. (1973). Conformity and anti–conformity among Americans and Chinese. *Journal of Social Psychology, 89,* 15–24.
Meier, A., & Edwards, J. (1974). Purpose in life test: Age and sex differences. *Journal of Clinical Psychology, 30,* 384–386.
Morojele, N. K., & Brooks, J. S. (2004). Sociodemographic, sociocultural, and individual predictors of reporting feelings of meaninglessness among South African adolescents. *Psychological Reports, 95,* 1271–1278.
Oishi, S., & Diener, E. (2003). Culture and well–being: The cycle of action, evaluation, and decision. *Personality and Social Psychology Bulletin, 29,* 939–949.
Padelford, B. L. (1974). Relationship between drug involvement and purpose in life. *Journal of Clinical Psychology, 30,* 303–305.
Paloutzian, R. F. (1981). Purpose in life and value changes following conversion. *Journal of Personality and Social Psychology, 41*(6), 1153–1160.
Paloutzian, R. F., & Ellison, C. W. (1982). Loneliness, spiritual well–being, and quality of life. In L. A. Peplau, & D. Perlman (Eds.), *Loneliness: A Sourcebook of Current Theory, Research, and Therapy*. New York: Wiley.
Pan, J. Y., Wong, D. F. K., Joubert, L., & Chan, C. L. W. (2008). The protective function of meaning of life on life satisfaction among Chinese students in Australia and Hong Kong: A cross–cultural comparative study. *Journal of American College Health, 57*(2), 221–231.
Pearson, P. R., & Sheffield, B. F. (1974). Purpose in life and the Eysenck personality inventory. *Journal of Clinical Psychology, 30,* 562–564.
Pizzolato, J. E., Brown, E. L., & Kanny, M. A. (2011). Purpose plus: Supporting youth purpose, control, and academic achievement. *New Directions for Youth Development, 132,* 75–88.
Putnam, R. (2007). E Pluribus Unum: Diversity & community in the twenty–first century. The Johan Skytte prize lecture. *Scandinavian political studies, 30,* 137–174.
Reker, G. T. (1977). The purpose in life test in an inmate population: An empirical investigation. *Journal of Clinical Psychology, 33*(3), 688–693.
Ross, C. E., & Mirowsky, J. (2009). Neighborhood disorder, subjective alienation, and distress. *Journal of Health and Social Behavior, 50,* 49–64.
Ryff, C. D. (1995). Psychological well–being in adulthood. *Current Directions in Psychological Science, 4*(4), 99–104.
Ryff, C. D., Keyes, C. L. M., & Hughes, D. L. (2003). Status inequalities, perceived discrimination, and eudaimonic well–being: Do the challenges of minority life hone purpose and growth? *Journal of Health and Social Behavior, 44,* 275–291.

Ryff, C. D., & Singer, B. (2008). Know thyself and become what you are: A eudaimonic approach to psychological well–being. *Journal of Happiness Studies, 9,* 13–39.

Salmela-Aro, K., & Nurmi, J-E (1997). Goal contents, well–being and life context during the transition to university: A longitudinal study. *International Journal of Behavioral Development, 20,* 471–491.

Scannell, E. D., Allen, F. C. L., & Burton, J. (2002). Meaning in life and positive and negative well–being. *North American Journal of Psychology, 4*(1), 93–111.

Schlesinger, S., Susman, M., & Koenigsberg, J. (1990). Self–esteem and purpose in life: A comparative study of women alcoholics. *Journal of Alcohol and Drug Education, 36,* 127–141.

Schwartz, C. E., Keyl, P. M., Marcum, J. P., & Bode, R. (2009). Helping others shows differential benefits on health and well–being for male and female teens. *Journal of Happiness Studies, 10,* 431–448.

Seligman, M. E. P. (2002). *Authentic happiness: Using the new positive psychology to realize your potential for lasting fulfillment.* New York: Free.

Shek, D. T. L., Hong, E.W., & Cheung, M. Y. P.(1987). The Purpose in Life Questionnaire in a Chinese context. *The Journal of Psychology, 121*(1), 77–83.

Simmons, D. D. (1980). Purpose in life and the three aspects of valuing. *Journal of Clinical Psychology, 36*(4), 921–922.

Soderstrom, D., & Wright, E. W. (1977). Religious orientation and meaning in life. *Journal of Clinical Psychology, 33*(1), 65–68.

Steger, M. F., Frazier, P., Oishi, S., & Kaler, M. (2006). The meaning in life questionnaire: Assessing the presence of and search for meaning in life. *Journal of Counseling Psychology, 53*(1), 80–91.

Steger, M. F., Kashdan, T. B., Oishi, S. (2007). Being good by doing good: Daily eudaimonic activity and well–being. *Journal of Research in Personality, 42,* 22–42.

Steger, M. F., Kashdan, T. B., Sullivan, B. A., & Lorentz, D. (2008a). Understanding the search for meaning in life: Personality, cognitive style, and the dynamic between seeking and experiencing meaning. *Journal of Personality, 76,* 199–228.

Steger, M. F., Kawabata, Y., Shimai, S., & Otake, K. (2008b). The meaningful life in Japan and the United States: Levels and correlates of meaning in life. *Journal of Research in Personality, 42,* 660–678.

Stillman, T. F., Baumeister, R. F., Lambert, N., Crescioni, A. W., DeWall, C. N., & Fincham, F. D. (2009). Alone and without purpose: Life loses meaning following social exclusion. *Journal of Experimental Social Psychology, 45,* 686–94.

Umberson, D., & Gove, W. (1989). Parenthood and psychological well–being: Theory, measurement, and stage in the life course. *Journal of Family Issues, 10,* 440–462.

Yang, K. S. (1981). The formation and change of Chinese personality: A cultural ecological perspective. *ACTA Psychologica Taiwanica, 23,* 39–55.

Yarnell, T. D. (1971). Purpose in life test: Further correlates. *Journal of Individual Psychology, 27,* 76–79.

Yeagar, D., & Bundick, M. (2009). The role of purposeful work goals in promoting meaning in life and in schoolwork during adolescence. *Journal of Adolescent Research, 24*(4), 423–452.

Zeitchik, G. (2000). The construct validity of the purpose in life test: Quantifying Victor Frankl's "will to meaning" (unpublished doctoral dissertation, Garden City, NY, Adelphi University). *Dissertation Abstracts International, 61,* 09B 5049.

Zika, S., & Chamberlain, K. (1987). Relation of hassles and personality to subjective well–being. *Journal of Personality and Social Psychology, 53,* 155–162.

Chapter 8
Exemplar Research

Definitional Matters

As is evident in preceding discussions, the purpose construct has been examined in a variety of ways and from a range of perspectives. Diary methods (e.g. Inhelder and Piaget 1958; Steger et al. 2007), intervention studies (e.g. Burrow 2012; Dik et al. 2011; King et al. 2006; Pizzolato et al. 2011), document reviews (e.g. Mariano and Vaillant 2012), survey research (e.g. Crumbaugh and Maholick 1969; Meirer and Edwards 1974; Ryff 1989; Schmutte and Ryff 1997), and interview methodologies (e.g. Bronk et al. 2010; Damon 2008; Yeagar and Bundick 2009) have all been used to examine purpose and related meaning constructs (See Chap. 2, Measuring Purpose, for a more complete discussion of measures and methods for studying the purpose construct). Use of these varied approaches has yielded significant insight into the nature and prevalence of more typical and deficient forms of purpose; however, while these methods all have notable strengths, none is able to provide a clear picture of complete or nearly complete purpose development (Damon and Colby in press). To gain this understanding, exemplar studies are needed.

The exemplar methodology is a sample selection technique that involves the intentional selection of individuals, groups, or entities that exemplify the construct of interest in a highly developed manner (Bronk 2012a, b). In using the exemplar methodology, researchers deliberately select and study a sample of individuals or entities that exhibit a particular characteristic in an intense or highly developed way. Accordingly, exemplar methodologies feature participants who are rare, not from the perspective of the characteristics they exhibit, but in the highly developed way they demonstrate those particular characteristics. Exemplar studies of youth purpose, for example, feature individuals who demonstrate intense, all-encompassing commitments to personally meaningful aspirations.

The exemplar methodology has most commonly been used to explore ethical constructs including the development of morality (Colby and Damon 1992; MacRenato 1995; Mastain 2007; Matsuba and Walker 2005), spirituality (King 2010), altruism (Oliner and Oliner 1988), environmental activism (Pratt 2011), care (Hart and Fegley 1995; Walker and Frimer 2007), and bravery (Walker and Frimer 2007). It makes sense that a methodology focused on ideal states would be used to

K. C. Bronk, *Purpose in Life*, DOI 10.1007/978-94-007-7491-9_8,

study positive, moral constructs, but it need not be limited to this area of study. The exemplar methodology can be used to gain an understanding of the complete or nearly complete growth of any developmental construct.

Not only *can* the approach be used more widely in studies of human development, but as well it *should* be used more widely. An understanding of the full range of growth requires not only information about deficient and typical growth, as provided by existing methodologies, but also about the leading edge of development, as provided by the exemplar methodology (Damon and Colby in press). Combining conclusions from exemplar research with findings from studies featuring more typical individuals yields a comprehensive and detailed understanding of the full spectrum of development required for a more complete account of human growth.

Exemplars represent the upper ends of development with regards to the constructs they exemplify, but in other ways, they are unlikely to differ significantly from more typical individuals (Bronk 2012a). In other areas, their development is likely to be average or even retarded, and because exemplars are not particularly far removed from more typical individuals, what we learn from them can shed important light on more typical developmental processes. In Colby and Damon's (1992) study of moral exemplars, for instance, the authors note "Great moral acts… spring from the same sources as lesser ones" (p. 4). In other words, exemplars follow the same developmental path as more typical individuals; they just advance further. They reveal a highly developed form of the construct of interest, meaning that whenever more typical individuals become capable of doing something new, they trace the steps of where the exemplars have already been (Damon and Colby in press). Accordingly, the study of exemplars reveals important information about the likely developmental trajectory of more typical individuals.

From a methodological standpoint, the exemplar approach has historically been situated within the broader case study tradition. Gordon Allport (1962), one of the early proponents of case study methodologies, argued that idiographic methods were useful for countering the "thinness" of nomothetic methods. Case study research allows for a highly detailed, contextual analysis of complex issues, objects, and individuals. Yin (1984) defined case study research as an empirical method of inquiry that investigates a contemporary phenomenon within its real-life context; it is useful when the boundaries between phenomenon and context are not clearly evident; and it relies on multiple sources of evidence. Because case studies are often used to address *why* and *how* questions, they can be exploratory, explanatory, or descriptive in nature (Tellis 1997). Researchers have used the case study method for many years across a variety of disciplines, but social scientists, in particular, have made wide use of this qualitative research method to examine the growth of individuals in context.

While the exemplar methodology has historically been used in qualitative studies, it can also be used in quantitative research. In fact, many recent exemplar studies have included larger samples of exemplars and have featured quantitative research designs (e.g. Matsuba and Walker 2004; Walker and Frimer 2007).

Whether using the exemplar methodology to conduct qualitative or quantitative research, it is important to thoughtfully consider how exemplars are selected. Effective exemplar studies typically feature the use of nomination criteria that are used to qualify individuals as exemplars (Bronk 2012a). Nomination criteria may outline experiences, attributes, awards, or behavioral manifestations indicative of high levels of development in a particular area. Nomination criteria are typically shared with nominators, often experts in the area, who use them to identify potential exemplars.

Aristotle was one of the earliest thinkers to consider the importance of the exemplar methodology. In *Nicomachean Ethics* he wrote, "We approach the subject of practical wisdom by studying the persons to whom we attribute it" (1962, 6.5 1140a25). Put another way, to understand how a complex construct functions and develops, it makes sense to examine it in the lives of individuals who exhibit it in a particularly consistent and highly developed manner. Along these same lines, Maslow (1971) was one of the earliest scholars to actually employ the exemplar methodology, though he, like Aristotle, never called it that. Interested in understanding how people achieve self-actualization, Maslow focused his study on individuals who he believed were fully self-actualized. Development, he claimed, "is learning to grow and learning what to grow toward" (p. 169). Therefore, if we want to learn about what is possible with regards to personally meaningful aspirations, we should study individuals with a highly developed sense of purpose in life.

Youth Purpose Exemplars

Researchers at the Stanford Center on Adolescence conducted a five-year, longitudinal study of adolescent purpose exemplars (Damon 2008). Under the direction of principal investigator William Damon, researchers selected a sample of adolescents who demonstrated intense commitments to various purposes in life. The young people were interviewed three times over a five-year period that spanned much of adolescence and emerging adulthood. Interviews were conducted approximately every two and a half years and, in typical case-study style, lasted roughly three hours each. The youths' parents and colleagues or peers were also interviewed.

Nomination criteria, which were largely based on the definition of purpose, included the following: youth purpose exemplars,

- demonstrated a commitment to a long-term aim,
- engaged in working toward their far-horizon aspiration,
- devised realistic plans for continuing to work toward this goal in the future,
- believed that their long-term aims were deeply, personally meaningful,
- and, were motivated to achieve their long-term, personally meaningful aims at least in part because doing so allowed them to have an impact on the broader world (Bronk 2005, 2008, 2011, 2012b, pp. 83–84).

Expert youth workers in a variety of areas, including music education, sports, religious education, community service, and extracurricular activities, applied the nomination criteria to identify potential purpose exemplars. Members of the research team contacted each of the potential exemplars and confirmed, in a brief screening interview, that each met the stated nomination criteria.

The resulting sample included youth committed to a wide range of activities and interests. Slightly more than half the group was dedicated to a social cause, including raising money to build wells in Africa, supporting cancer research, sharing important news events through journalism, promoting adolescent health, and preserving the environment. The other five were devoted to making progress toward other aims, including creating jazz music, promoting conservative political ideals, creating new technologies, and serving God.

The resulting data from these interviews are at once far-reaching and highly detailed. Analyses of the data have yielded insight into what the leading edge of the development of purpose looks like in practice. The data have been analyzed from a variety of perspectives, and findings shed light on the characteristics of purposeful youth, the relationship between purpose development and identity formation, and the development of purpose over time. A summary of the main findings from each analysis is included below.

Characteristics of Purposeful Youth (Bronk 2008**)** The first analysis of the youth purpose exemplar data identifies defining characteristics of young purpose exemplars. This analysis included a comparison sample of non-purposeful youth, who were matched with the purpose exemplars for age, sex, and ethnicity. They were included to discern if the characteristics that emerged among the purposeful sample were indeed particular to this group of young people.

Results suggest that the youth purpose exemplars do share certain features that distinguish them from other youth, including vitality, openness, focus, and humility (Bronk 2005). Vitality represents a psychological construct with emotional and cognitive components. It is marked by feelings of positivity or optimism, enthusiasm and energy, and a belief that one is eager to act and capable of doing so effectively (Nix et al. 1999; Ryan and Frederick 1997). Purpose exemplars consistently exhibited three different forms of vitality, including positive energy and a general busyness, a positive or optimistic view of the future, and confidence in their ability to be effective and have an impact. Additionally, the exemplars demonstrated different facets of authentic or intellectual humility (Roberts 2012).

While it might not be surprising to find that the exemplars were particularly busy and maybe not even surprising to learn that they were optimistic and efficacious, given their commitments, it was surprising to find that they were humble (Bronk 2008). Humility was the most striking and theoretically interesting characteristic to emerge from this grounded theory analysis of purpose exemplars.

According to Tangney (2000, 2002), one of the most widely cited writers on humility, there are four cognitive features of authentic humility. First, authentic humility means having an accurate, not over- or under-estimated sense of one's abilities and achievements, including having an accurate assessment of one's shortcomings, imperfections, limitations, and gaps in knowledge. Second, authentic humility is associated with being open to new ideas and to contradictory information and advice. In other words, rather than ignoring perspectives that do not align with their own, humble individuals tend to embrace these perspectives and use them to develop and improve their ideas. Third, being humble means maintaining a relatively low self-focus. Tangney even refers to a "forgetting of the self." Finally, authentic humility entails appreciating the value of all things, as well as the many ways that people and things contribute to the broader world. Authentic humility, according to this definition, represents not a limitation, but instead a useful strength of character (Peterson and Seligman 2004).

Humility is not a characteristic typically associated with adolescents, especially not adolescents, such as the exemplars, who have earned recognition, often high-level, public recognition, for their accomplishments. Though humility was not intentionally probed in interviews with either the sample of purposeful or non-purposeful youth, 107 instances of the construct emerged from the purposeful sample and only twelve instances were evident among the non-purposeful sample. Each of these manifestations of humility was categorized into one of the following humility subcodes: (1) openness (e.g. being open to learning and growing, being open-minded, and seeking new perspectives), (2) the accurate assessment of strengths and weaknesses, (3) an appreciation for others' contributions, and (4) a low self-focus.

Openness Among the non-purposeful youth, only four instances of openness appeared, but among the purposeful youth, 65 instances of openness emerged. In fact, this was the most common manifestation of humility among the purpose exemplars. Each of the exemplars demonstrated some form of openness, but its role and form varied. Forms of openness included intellectual curiosity, an appreciation for opposing perspectives, and open-mindedness. Interestingly, each of the forms of openness supported the youths' pursuit of purpose in a slightly different way. Being open helped the youth discover purposes, as they remained receptive to potentially significant aspirations, and pursue purposes over time, as they remained interested in finding new ways of making progress toward personally meaningful aims.

However, had the youth with purpose only been open, without also being focused, they likely would not have accomplished much. An unmoored person can easily be swayed from one direction to another without making much forward progress. The purpose exemplars, however, accomplished quite a bit, and their ability to consistently balance a sharp focus with an inquisitive openness allowed them to do this. In practice, this meant they allowed their personally meaningful aspiration to serve as a compass of sorts, guiding them in a consistent direction. At the same time, they remained open to reinterpreting what their aspirations meant to them and how they could most effectively reach them. As situations changed and new information and resources became available, often in conjunction with the normative transitions associated with adolescence and emerging adulthood (e.g. leaving for college, starting work, etc), the youth purpose exemplars altered the way they made progress toward their personally meaningful aspirations. For instance, during high school, a young woman honored her commitment to serving God by obeying her parents, attending church, and meditating on the Bible. When she went to college she lost contact with her religious community and no longer lived with her parents, so she served God by working hard in school so she could eventually pursue a career that would allow her to do the work she believed God intended her to do. She remained focused on her ultimate aim, but she was open to working toward it in different ways as her life circumstances changed.

Accurate Assessment of Personal Strengths and Weaknesses The second manifestation of humility that emerged among the youth purpose exemplars was the ability to reflect on and accurately assess their personal strengths and weaknesses. Each of the exemplars and less than half of the non-purposeful youth either spoke directly about their strengths and weaknesses or described incidences that revealed that personal assessments had taken place. For the purpose exemplars, approximately one fifth of the humility quotations were categorized into this sub-code (22 of 107), while for the non-purposeful sample, only seven quotations were categorized accordingly. Therefore, while this manifestation of humility was relatively rare among the non-purposeful sample, it was fairly common among the exemplars. They frequently told stories that signaled awareness of their capacities as well as their shortcomings. In one case, a young woman committed to working in healthcare administration to reported that at the beginning of college she had avoided economics courses. Though she thought an understanding of economics might be useful in a general sense, it did not appear to be necessary for the medical career she was pursuing, and economics was a difficult course on campus. Toward the end of her sophomore year, she came to realize that healthcare and economics are intricately intertwined. In fact, an understanding of economics was particularly important in the line of work she planned to pursue. Accordingly, not only did she need to take several economics courses, but she also ended up pursuing a masters degree in business administration along with her medical degree. She realized at least two shortcomings here. First, she recognized that economics did not come easily to her, and second, she realized that she was wrong to think she could avoid the learning about the field. She acknowledged these shortcomings, but she did not give into them. Instead, she worked hard to overcome them. This was a typical pattern of behavior among the other youth purpose exemplars as well.

Being able to recognize one's strengths and weaknesses is essential to any goal pursuit, and purpose is no exception. A purpose in life represents an enduring, long-term aim, and as such it may be particularly important for purposeful individuals to recognize their own strengths and weaknesses. If they are to make progress toward their purposeful aims, they need to know where their weaknesses lie so they can recognize when they require assistance, instruction, and when they should be willing to alter their course of action. Likewise, they need to know where their strengths lie so they know when to take the lead and when to remain firm in their beliefs and practices. In this way, this important manifestation of humility likely facilitated the purpose exemplars pursuit of their personal aspirations.

Appreciation for Others' Contributions The third aspect of humility that surfaced among this sample was an appreciation for the value of all things. One non-purposeful youth made a comment coded this way, and fourteen of the purpose exemplars' quotations were categorized into this sub-code. The purposeful youth recognized the helpful roles that others played in their own lives and in their pursuit of purpose.

This manifestation of humility was particularly evident in the young environmentalist. She noted that a prestigious Environmental Protection Agency award she won was not really her award alone. It belonged instead to a cadre of family members, friends, and mentors who had helped her along the way. Accordingly, she was quick to share the spotlight and honor those who had aided in the broader effort.

Being able to appreciate the contributions of others likely helped the young people make progress toward their ultimate aims in a variety of ways, but perhaps most importantly, it made others more willing to work with and mentor them. When people take all the credit for success, others are not particularly keen to assist them, but when people are willing to share credit and to recognize others' contributions, people are much happier to help. In this way, the propensity to recognize others' contributions likely facilitated the pursuit of purpose in that it helped the youth garner help and support from friends, colleagues, and mentors.

Low Self-focus Another, way the purpose exemplars likely endeared themselves to others was by maintaining a low self-focus. None of the non-purposeful youth and three of the purpose exemplars made comments indicative of a low self-focus, making this the least common manifestation of purpose to emerge from both samples. One way the purpose exemplars demonstrated this facet of humility was by focusing not on their own accomplishments, but instead on the importance of the cause. Remaining focused on the ultimate aim, rather than on their own achievements in pursuit of that aim, likely endeared the purposeful youth to potentially helpful like-minded peers and mentors, thereby increasing available sources of support for the ongoing development of purpose. Maintaining a low self-focus likely also helped the exemplars weather setbacks. Failures and hinderances could be viewed as part of the purposeful pursuit rather than as a characteristic of the individual.

It is noteworthy that humility, in all four forms, spontaneously emerged as a consistent, defining characteristic of each of the purpose exemplars and of none of the non-purposeful youth. We cannot conclude from this analysis whether it is the case that purpose spurs the development of humility or if humility encourages the development of purpose or if a third factor contributes to the growth of both constructs. However, regardless of the direction of causality, it is clear that humility, at least in some cases, can play an important role in supporting purpose and together—purpose and humility—can position youth to develop in positive directions.

Chapter 3 (The Role of Purpose in Optimal Human Functioning) outlines the many ways that purpose contributes to positive youth development, but it is not entirely clear how humility fosters healthy growth. Templeton (1995, 1997) has theorized that the openness dimension of humility facilitates intellectual growth, and arrogance serves as a significant barrier to the acquisition of new knowledge. Remaining open, allows individuals to seek out new information and learn more about the things that interest them. In the case of humble purpose exemplars, these individuals remained open to learning about their personal aspirations, and this likely helped them make progress toward their ultimate aims. Being open to learning and growing allowed the young people to glean a variety of important lessons that helped them find and maintain their purposes and that will likely position them to learn other important life lessons, as well. Building practical knowledge is an important step in progressing toward purpose and positive youth development.

Another way that humility helped the exemplars pursue their personal aspirations and contributed to their positive development was through increasing the likelihood that these youth would establish relationships with mentors and like-minded peers. Each of the purpose exemplars reported having long-term mentoring relationships characterized by frequent interaction with adults who helped them learn more about and pursue their respective interests. Mentors were far less common among the non-purposeful youth and when they were present, the relationships tended to be brief and less impactful. Similarly, rather than working alone toward their aims, purpose exemplars sought out peers who shared and supported their interests. Working with supportive others not only served to decrease the chances that they would lose interest over time, but also decreased the odds that they would veer off their positive developmental trajectory over time. An openness to learning, an appreciation for others' contributions, and an ability to accurately assess their shortcomings represent characteristics that likely made the exemplars desirable protégées, attractive friends, and valued colleagues. With the help of prosocial mentors and supportive peers and colleagues, the exemplars were better positioned to discover and maintain purposes over time. The role like-minded peers and mentors play in supporting purpose is elaborated upon in Chap. 5 (Origins and supports for purpose).

Purpose Development and Identity Formation (Bronk 2011)

The second analysis of the youth purpose exemplar data focused on the relationship between purpose development and identity formation. Chapter 4 (Purpose across the Lifespan) provides a fuller discussion of the role purpose plays in healthy identity development, but briefly, Erikson (1968) argued that under optimal conditions young people develop a coherent and relatively stable sense of identity that includes making commitments to personally meaningful values, beliefs, and plans. In other words, purpose can represent an important outcome of healthy identity development. More contemporary research confirms that youth explore and commit to purposes at roughly the same time that they explore and commit to identities (Burrow et al. 2010). Not only do purpose and identity develop at roughly the same time, but they also share a focus on personally meaningful beliefs and aims. However, despite their concomitant appearance in the lifespan, and despite their shared focus, purpose and identity represent distinct constructs. In short, identity refers to who one hopes to become and purpose to what one hopes to accomplish (Bronk 2011; Erikson 1968).

Again, as discussed in Chap. 4 (Purpose across the Lifespan), a growing body of empirical research suggests that purpose and identity serve as reinforcing constructs, whereby growth in one facilitates growth in the other (Côté 1996, 1997).

It has been theorized that discovering purpose may help individuals resolve their identity "crisis" by offering them a meaningful aim to which they can direct time, energy, and effort (Burrow and Hill 2011), and resolving an identity "crisis" may result in the development of new assets, capabilities, or talents, which are likely to facilitate the growth of purpose (Burrow et al. 2010).

While Erikson (1968) and others have suggested that identity and purpose are related constructs, little empirical research has focused on *how* they function together. Therefore, this second analysis sought to clarify the nature of the relationship between these two hallmarks of healthy adolescent development. Results suggest that purpose helps foster identity formation, that identity formation deepens purposeful commitments and, in this way, purpose and identity, at least among some youth, can support and reinforce one another.

Purpose Fosters Identity Formation Pursuing purpose influenced the way the exemplars viewed themselves with regard to the broader social world and the way they viewed themselves over time. Côté and Levine (2002) refer to these varied perspectives on the self as social and ego identities respectively, and in significant ways, pursuing purpose fostered growth in both areas.

With regards to social identity formation, working toward personally meaningful aspirations allowed the exemplars to see how they fit in and could be of use to the broader world. For instance, the young environmentalist explained how her work helped her find her "place in the world.... To have found where I feel like I'm doing something for the place that I live, which is my world. Feeling like this is where I'm supposed to be, this is what I'm supposed to be doing. I'm benefitting these people... in the work I do. I'm helping someone else because of the abilities I have.... These are things that I have to offer this world" (Bronk 2011, p. 37). The other exemplars made similar statements that underscored the important avenue purpose provided for finding their places in the world beyond-themselves.

With regards to ego identity development, having a purpose helped the exemplars establish an enduring sense of self framed by their aspirations. Ego identity refers to a "vital sense of one's continuity and sameness" (Côté and Levine 2002, p. 182) and a stable sense of who one is and what one believes in. Evidence of the central role of purpose in the establishment of an ego identity emerged when the exemplars identified themselves by their purposeful commitments. For example, the youth purpose exemplars regularly identified themselves by their purposes. For example, the religious exemplar noted, "I'm a Christian, because I'm dedicated to doing what God wants me to do" (Bronk 2011, p. 37).

This finding highlights at least one potential mechanism for the way purpose fosters positive youth development. Finding that purpose provides a personally meaningful opportunity for social and ego identity development lends support to theoretical claims that purpose can serve as an identity-related resource (Burrow and Hill 2011; Burrow et al. 2010; Côté and Levine 2002). The identity capital model proposes that tangible and intangible resources support optimal identity formation and individualization (Côté 2002). Committing to a purpose in life may serve as an important intangible, identity-related resource, as discovering purpose offered the exemplars a personally meaningful direction toward which to dedicate their energy and focus (Burrow and Hill 2011).

Identity Formation Reinforces Purpose Development Pursuing purpose fostered identity formation, and advances in identity formation reinforced commitments to purpose. As others identified youth with their personal aspirations, the exemplars' purposeful commitments intensified. The young environmentalist noted that her friends referred to her as a "tree hugger". She took pride in this nick name, and it inspired he to intensify her committment to preserving the natural world.

As Erikson (1968) noted, the development of purpose tends to precede the formation of identity, so it is not surprising that this study found that identity formation did not spur purpose development, but instead supported its ongoing growth. Bem's self-perception theory suggests that individuals infer their attitudes in part by observing their own behavior (1972). It seems likely that the exemplars' continued involvement led them to infer a deep connection to the activities in which they were engaged. Individuals close to the exemplars further confirmed this association by identifying the exemplars with their involvement, and in this way, the exemplars' developing sense of identity served to deepen their commitment to their purposes.

Purpose and Identity Are Overlapping Constructs Given that purpose development fostered identity formation and that identity formation supported the ongoing development of purpose, we can conclude that purpose and identity are reinforcing constructs, and in the case of the purpose exemplars, overlapping ones, as well. While purpose and identity may be related, but distinct constructs for more typical individuals, they shared highly similar characteristics among the exemplars. Put otherwise, who individuals with highly developed forms of purpose are appears to be largely defined by the personally meaningful aims they hope to accomplish.

This conclusion has implications for our understanding of how the youth purpose construct functions with regards to identity formation. The emerging model of purpose and identity growth, based on these findings, appears to resemble the model of moral identity. For moral exemplars an individual's sense of self and moral concerns are closely aligned, while for more typical individuals, identity and moral concerns function somewhat independently (Blasi 1984; Colby and Damon 1992). Similarly, we know that for purpose exemplars, purposeful concerns and identity are closely aligned as well, and that for youth without purpose, identity and purpose (or the lack thereof) are independent of one another. Research finds that youth can be divided into one of three categories based on their level of purposeful commitment: those who meet all the criteria for purpose; those who meet some of the criteria for purpose; and those who meet none of the criteria for purpose (Bronk et al. 2010). Youth who meet only some of the criteria for purpose would be expected to demonstrate a level of alignment between purpose and identity growth that falls somewhere between the full alignment of purpose exemplars and the complete lack of alignment evident among youth without purpose, but empirical research is needed to confirm this emerging theory.

Youth Purpose Development (Bronk 2012b)

As discussed in Chap. 5 (origins of and supports for purpose) the third and final analysis conducted on the purpose exemplar data focused on gaining a deeper understanding of the way purpose is discovered and changes or evolves over time (Bronk 2012b). Based on the definition of purpose, we would expect to find that an individual's personal aspirations are enduring and relatively stable. Findings in this analysis confirm that purpose exemplars' aims are lasting, at least across the busy stages of adolescence and emerging adulthood. Results further conclude that commitment serves as an important organizing structure in the growth of personal aspirations. Accordingly, this study posits a theory of purpose development based on processes tied to commitment, including: initiating commitment, sustaining commitment, escalating commitment, and evolving commitment.

Initiating Commitments During childhood, the young purpose exemplars got involved in activities that would later take on a more significant role in their lives. For instance, one exemplar noted that her commitment to cancer research stemmed from her experience selling daffodils at age six to raise money for the American Cancer Society.

As discussed in Chap. 5 (Origins of and Support for Purpose) the early activities that youth select are influenced by where they grew up and by the opportunities available to them. For example, the environmental exemplar grew up in rural Texas. She became interested in environmental work when she witnessed her dad pouring motor oil into the soil near her home. She worried about the impact this might have on the family's drinking water, which came from a nearby underground well. When given the opportunity to carry out a 4-H project, she decided to investigate the environmental impact of oil and to make available an easier way for farmers living in rural areas, like her dad, to safely dispose of their excess motor oil. Growing up in the country shaped her commitment to environmental activism in important ways.

Sustaining Commitment Deriving pleasure and a deep sense of meaning from engagement in their purposeful commitments coupled with the ability to devise useful strategies for overcoming challenges (e.g. thriving on challenge, focusing on prosocial motivators, remaining confident in an eventual solution, and using novel tactics to solve old problems) helped the exemplars sustain their commitments over time. The youth purpose exemplars thrived on being engaged in purposeful activities. In discussing her passion for cancer work, for instance, one exemplar told the following story,

> A couple of weeks ago I was at the Foundation until like 3 a.m. on a Friday night. And like Friday night is when, you know, people are out whatever having fun, but because I just like I loved it so much…. Other things were secondary because I really, really felt like this is what I want to be doing… and that made me stay there until 3 a.m.. (Bronk 2012b, p. 89).

Many young people find activities they enjoy, but particular to the exemplars was the ability to use their talents and skills to fill personally valued social needs. For instance, the journalist shared this relevant story, "[I recently read a New York Times article about] a concealed weapon law that's allowed hundreds of criminals who have confessed or pled no contest to felonies to get firearms. I can't help but feel that I've got ideas and I've got resources where I can help solve some of these problems, so why wouldn't I try?" (Bronk 2012b, p. 90). Finding ways of applying special skills and capacities in service of personally significant social needs is the essence of purpose (Damon 2008).

We can conclude from these findings that the exemplars' initial involvement tended to be relatively minor in nature. However, once the exemplars became involved, they discovered that their talents made them particularly well suited to the work and knowing that they were able to help address an important social need helped instill the activity with a growing sense of personal meaningfulness.

Escalating Commitments Consequently, their committments grew over time. While involvement tended to increase and decrease depending on the other things going on in the exemplars' lives, on the whole levels of commitment rose over the course of adolescence and emerging adulthood. Initially commitment grew in response to positive feedback, and over time, it intensified as a result of supportive relationships with like-minded peers and mentors.

Positive feedback played an important role, especially early on, in deepening the young people's commitments, though what constituted positive feedback varied based on the individual. For some of the exemplars, positive feedback took the form of recognition for their talents and for others it represented small successes in pursuit of their aims.

Over time, positive feedback and recognition became less important in supporting the growth of purpose, and the support of like-minded peers and mentors became increasingly significant. Each of the exemplars noted that initially their friends did not share, and in some cases even opposed, their purposeful interests. That the purpose exemplars remained committed to their aims in spite of this is noteworthy, as adolescence is typically marked by a strong desire to fit in. The way the exemplars dealt with this was by finding new groups of peers who shared their interests. In some instances the exemplars discovered existing groups of like-minded peers, and in other cases they had to create these groups, but in the end all of the exemplars ended up surrounding themselves with individuals who shared and supported their personal aspirations. For instance, the adolescent health advocate was well aware of the lack of support among peers at her high school for her efforts to curb teen smoking, so she had to seek out a group of individuals who shared her passion. "I think a lot of [my commitment's growth over time had] to do with finding other young people, like with the tobacco movement, getting to the national scene. In 1998 I helped start the National Truth Campaign, but with 99 other youth from around the country.... There was a larger movement of people out there who also had the same belief" (Bronk 2012b, p. 97). Over time supportive peer relationships played an important role in fostering and intensifying the exemplars' commitments.

Not only were peers important, but mentors were as well. Learning how to act effectively in a new area required assistance from highly skilled and more knowledgeable individuals, and accordingly support from mentors also contributed to a deepened level of commitment among the purpose exemplars. The critical support role of like-minded peers and mentors is discussed in greater detail in Chap. 5 (Origins of and Supports for Purpose).

Evolving Commitments The adolescent and emerging adult stages of life feature multiple normative transitions, including transitions from middle school to high school and from high school to work or college. At each of these junctures the youth purpose exemplars, like other youth their age, met new people, encountered new experiences, and accessed new resources. Each transition offered opportunities for their commitments to evolve. One way this happened had to do with discovering new means of achieving old aims. Exemplars' aspirations remained consistent over time, but the way they worked toward those aims changed as their circumstances and contexts evolved.

Exemplars' aims also tended to broaden over time. For example, initially the well builder was singularly focused on raising money to build wells in third world countries. Over time, however, his interests expanded. By the time he was sixteen he had raised millions of dollars to help build hundreds of wells around the world. Media outlets began to highlight his work and others took notice of his accomplishments, and the youth began receiving scores of invitations to serve as a motivational speaker. His commitment to providing clean drinking water did not diminish, but he realized that he was now in a position to also encourage other people to reflect on the ways they could use their talents and skills to help others. Accordingly, his non-profit organization adopted a new, three-pronged mission: building clean water facilities, educating people on basic sanitation, and motivating others to use their capacities to effect personally meaningful change in the world.

Findings from the exemplar sample shed light on what the process of developing a purpose is likely to entail for more typical individuals, as well as for the exemplars. For instance, it is clear from the exemplar sample that context matters. All of the exemplars' purposes were influenced by the places they grew up. The issues relevant in their hometowns and the opportunities available there significantly impacted the nature of the purposes they pursued. Had they grown up in different places, they likely would have made different commitments or it is possible they would not have made any commitments at all. Context also influenced the way commitments were sustained over time. When environments featured supportive networks, purposes grew, and when they did not, commitments stalled. As is elaborated upon in Chap. 5 (Origins of and Supports for Purpose), supportive environments are key to the development and pursuit of purpose. While like-minded peers and caring mentors did not provide the motivation for purpose, they did guide the exemplars' search for purpose and they often made the exemplars aware of opportunities for deepening their involvement. This finding underscores the need for adults to remain vigilant of young peoples' budding interests and "sparks" (Benson 2008) and to take steps to connect youth with opportunities to become further engaged in these areas of deep personal interest (Damon 2008).

Second, according to the exemplars, they would not have discovered purposes in the areas they did had they not been engaged in particular activities areas early on, often as children. Accordingly, it is important to expose youth to potentially purposeful activities, including service, religious, familial, and work related activities as these kinds of activities could evolve into purposes. It is impossible to predict which activities, if any, are likely to inspire a lifelong commitment, but without exposure, the development of purpose seems doubtful. Initially, youth may not be overly excited about an activity, but through the course of their involvement they may discover a talent or skill that makes them well suited to helping fill a social need, and when that happens, purpose is likely to emerge. This theory is elaborated upon in Chap. 5 (Origins of and Supports for Purpose) and is supported by a significant body of service-learning research that concludes that even obligatory "volunteer work" can produce positive developmental outcomes (e.g. see Astin et al. 2000; Boss 1994; Miron et al. 2002; Raman and Pashupati 2002). However, rather than rushing from activity to activity, youth should be encouraged to participate in fewer activities, and to reflect more seriously on the impact of their involvement in each one (Fry 1998), as doing so is more likely to lead to serious considerations of special skills and personal meaningfulness (Bundick 2011).

Lastly, a sizable body of research finds that purpose contributes to positive youth development (Chap. 3, The Role of Purpose in Optimal Human Functioning, includes a fuller discussion of this relationship.), but few researchers have attempted to explain the mechanism through which this occurs. Those that have, generally point to the motivational pull of pursing purpose. Forming a prosocial commitment, they argue, draws young people along in a positive direction (Damon 2008; Moran 2009). Accordingly, a purpose in life serves as a beacon guiding youth through the potentially turbulent waters of the adolescent and emerging adult stages of life. While this certainly seems likely, it does not appear to be the whole story. Rather, in pursuit of their personal aspirations, the youth purpose exemplars unintentionally constructed positive developmental contexts for themselves, complete with caring mentors and supportive peer networks. These contexts supported not only their development of purpose, but also their positive growth more generally.

Exemplar research has yielded important conclusions in the broader field of positive psychology, and in the more particular study of youth purpose. Results from this line of inquiry reveal how highly developed forms of purpose commitment function, how they develop, and how they contribute to healthy growth. From these studies we glean what is possible, even if not common, regarding the development of purpose.

The exemplar methodology sheds light on the leading edge of development, and reveals the way highly developed forms of purpose function. Accordingly, use of this methodology allows us to predict what the path of purpose is likely to entail for individuals who discover a personally meaningful aim.

The methodology also reveals ways that parents, teachers, and other adults concerned about young people's well-being can effectively support the growth of purpose. For instance, adults should encourage youth to engage in potentially purposeful activities, connect youth with caring mentors and like-minded peers, and help youth take advantage of new resources to expand their commitments. To do this, of course, adults need to be cognizant of young people's budding purposes or "sparks" (Benson 2008).

It is evident that the exemplar approach to studying youth purpose has significantly expanded our understanding of the nature of the construct and the individuals who possess it. However, there is still more to learn from purpose exemplars. Additional analyses should be conducted on other samples of purpose exemplars to address a wider range of developmental questions. For instance, analyses should examine the role and function of purpose in later adult life stages. Following purpose exemplars from adolescence through midlife or even beyond would expand our understanding of the way this complex construct develops, grows, and changes over a much longer period of time. Further, a study of negative purpose exemplars is warranted to gain a deeper understanding of the way negative purposes develop and grow over time. Do these aims stem from the same sources as noble ones? Are ignoble purposes associated with any of the same positive developmental outcomes as more positive purposes? What sorts of early experiences are likely to foster the growth of immoral purposes? In what ways are the sources of support for ignoble and purposes similar and different? In sum, the exemplar methodology represents a useful approach to studying the purpose construct, and as such, continued work along these lines is needed.

However, the need for additional exemplar studies does not represent the only or even the most glaring hole in the existing research on purpose. Because psychologists have only relatively recently recognized the important ways purpose contributes to well-being, research on the construct is relatively new and remains far from complete. The following chapter (Chap. 9) discusses areas where additional research is needed and outlines ways studies might be designed to contribute to our growing understanding of purpose.

References

Allport, G. (1962). The general and the unique in psychological science. *Journal of Personality, 30,* 405–422.

Aristotle. (1962). *Nichomachean Ethics*. Englewood Cliffs, NJ: Prentice Hall.

Astin, A. W., Vogelgesang, L. J., Ikeda, E. K., & Yee, J. A. (2000). *How service learning affects students*. Los Angeles, CA: Higher Education Research Institute, UCLA.

Bem, D. (1972). Self-Perception Theory. In L. Berkowitz (Ed.), *Advances in Experimental Social Psychology (Vol. 6, pp. 1-62)*. New York, NY: Academic Press.

Benson, P. L. (2008). *Sparks: How parents can help ignite the hidden strengths of teenagers*. San Francisco: Jossey Bass.

Blasi, A. (1984). Moral identity: Its role in moral functioning. In W. M. Kurtines, & J. L. Gewirtz (Eds.), *Morality, moral behavior, and moral development* (pp. 129–139). New York, NY: Wiley.

Boss, J. A. (1994). The effect of community service work on the moral development of college ethics students. *Journal of Moral Education, 23*(2), 183–198.

Bronk, K. C. (2005). Portraits of purpose: A study examining the ways purpose contributes to positive youth development. (Doctoral Dissertation, Stanford University, 2006). *UMI ProQuest Digital Dissertations*, AAT 3187267.

Bronk, K. C. (2008). Humility among adolescent purpose exemplars. *Journal of Research on Character Education, 6*(1), 35–51.

Bronk, K. C. (2011). Portraits of purpose: The role of purpose in identity formation. *New Directions in Youth Development, 132,* 31–44.

Bronk, K. C. (2012a). The exemplar methodology: An approach to studying the leading edge of development. *Psychology of Well-Being: Theory, Research and Practice, 2*(5). DOI: 10.1186/2211-1522-2-5.

Bronk, K. C. (2012b). A grounded theory of youth purpose. *Journal of Adolescent Research, 27*: 78–109. http://dx.doi.org/10.1177/0743558411412958.

Bronk, K. C., Menon, J. L., & Damon, W. (2004). *Youth purpose: Conclusions from a working conference of leading scholars*. John Templeton Foundation Press.

Bronk, K. C., Finch, W. H., & Talib, T. (2010). Purpose in life among high ability adolescents. *High Ability Studies, 21*(2), 133–145.

Bundick, M. (2011). The benefits of reflecting on and discussing purpose in life in emerging adulthood. *New Directions for Youth Development, 132,* 89–103.

Burrow, A. (March 2012). *Beyond cross-sectional studies of youth purpose: Conclusions from the train study of purpose*. Paper presented at the 2012 biennial meeting of the Society for Research on Adolescence, Vancouver, Canada.

Burrow, A., & Hill, P. L. (2011). Purpose as a form of identity capital for positive youth adjustment. *Developmental Psychology, 47*(4), 1196–1206.

Burrow, A. L., O'Dell, A., & Hill, P. (2010). Profiles of a developmental asset: Youth purpose as a context for hope and well-being. *Journal of Youth and Adolescence, 39,* 1265–1273.

Colby, A., & Damon, W. (1992). *Some do care: Contemporary lives of moral commitment*. New York, NY: Free Press.

Côté, J. E. (1996). Sociological perspectives on identity formation: The culture-identity link and identity capital. *Journal of Adolescence, 19,* 417–428.

Côté, J. E. (1997). An empirical test of the identity capital model. *Journal of Adolescence, 20,* 577–597.

Côté, J. E. (2002). The role of identity capital in the transition to adulthood: The individualization thesis examined. *Journal of Youth Studies, 5*(2), 117–134.

Côté, J. E., & Levine, C. G. (2002). *Identity formation, agency, and culture: A social psychological synthesis*. Mahwah, NJ: Lawrence Erlbaum Associates.

Crumbaugh, J. C., & Maholick, L. T. (1969). *Manual of Instructions for the Purpose in Life test.* Munster, IN: Psychometric Affiliates.

Damon, W. (2008). *The path to purpose: Helping children find their calling in life*. New York, NY: Free Press.

Damon, W., & Colby, A. (in press). Why a true account of human development requires exemplar research. In K. Matsuba, P. E. King, & K. C. Bronk (Eds.), Exemplar methods and research: Quantitative and qualitative strategies for investigation. New Directions in Child and Adolescent Development.

Dik, B. J., Steger, M. F., Gibson, A., & Peisner, W. (2011). Make Your Work Matter: Development and pilot evaluations of a purpose-centered career education intervention. *New Directions for Youth Development, 132,* 59–73.

Erikson, E. H. (1968). *Identity: Youth and crisis*. New York, NY: Norton.

Fry, P. A. (1998). The development of personal meaning and wisdom in adolescence: A reexamination of moderating and consolidating factors and influences. In P. T. P. Wong (Ed.), *The human quest for meaning: A handbook of psychological research and clinical applications* (2nd ed.) (pp. 91–110). New York: Routledge.

Hart, D., & Fegley, S. (1995). Prosocial behavior and caring in adolescence: Relations to self-understanding and social judgment. *Child Development, 66,* 1346–1359.

Inhelder, B., & Piaget, J. (1958). *The growth of logical thinking from childhood to adolescence.* New York: Basic Books.

King, P. (March 2010). *Spiritual exemplars from around the world: An exploratory study of spiritual development among adolescents*. Paper presented at the 2010 biennial meeting of the Society for Research on Adolescence, Philadelphia, PA.

King, L. A., Hicks, J. A., & Krull, J., & Del Gaiso, A. K. (2006). Positive affect and the experience of meaning in life. *Journal of Personality and Social Psychology, 90,* 179–196.

MacRenato, S. W. (1995). *Experiences of moral commitment: A phenomenological study*. San Diego, CA: University of San Diego.

Mariano, J. M., & Vaillant, G. E. (2012). Purpose among the "Greatest Generation." *Journal of Positive Psychology*. DOI:10.1080/17439760.2012.686624.

Maslow, A. (1971). *The farther reaches of human nature*. New York: Viking Press.

Mastain, L. (2007). The lived experience of altruism as described by moral exemplars: A descriptive phenomenological study. *Dissertation Abstracts International*, DAI-B 67/12. (AAT 3246550).

Matsuba, M. K., & Walker, L. (2005). Young adult moral exemplars: The making of self through stories. *Journal of Research on Adolescence, 15*(3), 275–297.

Meier, A., & Edwards, H. (1974). Purpose-in-life Test: Age and sex differences. *Journal of Clinical Psychology, 30,* 384–386.

Miron, D., Moely, B. E., McFarland, M., & Mercer, S. (2002). Changes in college students' attitudes and intentions for civic involvement as a function of service-learning experiences. *Michigan Journal of Community Service Learning, 8*(2), 15–26.

Moran, S. (2009). Purpose: Giftedness in intrapersonal intelligence. *High Ability Studies, 20*(2), 143–159.

Nix, G. A., Ryan, R. M., Manly, J. B., & Deci, E. L. (1999). Revitalization through self-regulation: The effects of autonomous and controlled motivation on happiness and vitality. *Journal of Experimental Social Psychology, 35,* 266–284.

Oliner, S. P., & Oliner, M. P. (1988). *The altruistic personality: Rescuers of Jews in Nazi Europe: What Led Ordinary Men and Women to Risk their Lives on Behalf of Others?* New York: The Free Press.

Peterson, C., & Seligman, M. E. P. (2004). *Character strengths and virtues: A handbook of classification*. New York: Oxford University Press.

Pizzolato, J. E., Brown, E. L., & Kanny, M. A. (2011). Purpose plus: Supporting youth purpose, control, and academic achievement. *New Directions for Youth Development, 132,* 75–88.

Pratt, M. (2011). *Environmental memories of youth and adults: Identity and exemplar status predict story recall and level of detail*. Paper presented at the biennial meeting of the Society for Research on Child Development. Montreal, Canada.

Raman, P., & Pashupati, K. (2002). Turning good citizens into even better ones: The impact of program characteristics and motivations on service learning outcomes. *Journal of Nonprofit & Public Sector Marketing, 10*(2), 187–206.

Roberts, R. C. (June 24, 2012). What is it to be intellectually humble? Big Questions online. http://www.bigquestionsonline.com/content/what-it-beintellectually-humble. Accessed Aug. 7, 2013.

Ryan, R. M., & Frederick, C. M. (1997). On energy, personality and health: Subjective vitality as a dynamic reflection of well-being. *Journal of Personality, 65,* 529–565.

Ryff, C. D. (1989). Happiness is everything, or is it? Explorations on the meaning of psychological well-being. *Journal of Personality and Social Psychology, 57,* 1069–1081.

Schmutte, P. S., & Ryff, C. D. (1997). Personality and well-being: Reexamining methods and meanings. *Journal of Personality and Social Psychology, 73*(3), 549–559.

Steger, M. F., Kashdan, T. B., Oishi, S. (2007). Being good by doing good: Daily eudaimonic activity and well-being. *Journal of Research in Personality, 42,* 22–42.

Tangney, J. P. (2000). Humility: Theoretical perspectives, empirical findings, and directions for future research. *Journal of Social and Clinical Psychology, 19,* 70–82.

Tangney, J. P. (2002). Humility. In C. R. Snyder, & S. J. Lopez (Eds.), *Handbook of positive psychology* (pp. 411–419). New York: Oxford University Press.

Tellis, W. (July 1997). Introduction to case study [68 paragraphs]. *The Qualitative Report* [Online serial], *3*(2). Available: http://www.nova.edu/ssss/QR/QR3-2/tellis1.html. Accessed Aug. 7, 2013.

Templeton, J. M. (1995). *The humble approach*. New York: Continuum Publishing.

Templeton, J. M. (1997). *Worldwide laws of life*. Philadelphia: Templeton Foundation Colby, A. & Damon, W. (1992). *Some do care*. New York: The Free Press.
Walker, L. J., & Frimer, J. A. (2007). Moral personality of brave and caring exemplars. *Journal of Personality and Social Psychology, 93*(5), 845–860.
Yeager, D. S., & Bundick, M. (2009). The role of purposeful life goals in promoting meaning in life and schoolwork during adolescence. *Journal of Adolescent Research, 24*(4), 423–452.
Yin, R. (1984). *Case study research: Design and methods (1st ed.)*. Beverly Hills, CA: Sage Publishing.

Chapter 9
Future Directions for Purpose Research

In preparing to write this book, I scoured the purpose literature. I read hundreds of journal articles, book chapters, and books on the topic, and in the course of this deep and broad review, it became clear that much has been learned about purpose—what it is, how it can be assessed, its role in optimal human functioning, its developmental trajectory, how it begins, how it can be supported, the different forms it takes, and what it looks like in its fully developed form; however, there is still much to learn. Discussed here are some of the particularly significant omissions in the research.

Survey Measure of Purpose

One of the most glaring holes in the study of purpose has to do with research tools. To grow the body of research on the purpose construct, measurement tools that can easily and inexpensively assess the construct are needed. There is great diversity in the measurement tools currently available to assess purpose and closely related constructs. A wide range of survey measures has also been used (e.g. Purpose in Life test, PIL, Crumbaugh and Maholick 1964; Scales of Psychological Well-being Purpose sub-scale, Ryff and Keyes 1995). However, none of the existing survey measures assesses all dimensions of purpose.

As discussed in greater detail in the Chap. 1 (Introduction and Definition), a purpose in life represents an enduring intention to accomplish something that is both personally meaningful and at the same time leads to engagement with some aspect of the world beyond-the-self (Damon 2008; Damon et al. 2003). This definition highlights four components of the purpose construct. First, purpose represents a far-horizon goal. Individuals identify a personally meaningful aim toward which they hope to make progress. Second, commitment to purpose is underscored by active engagement as individuals invest time, energy, and resources to making progress toward their purposes. Third, one's purpose in life is highly personally meaningful. Finally, a purpose represents a desire to make a difference in the broader world. While the first three components are measured by most existing surveys of purpose, this last one is not. In fact, no existing measure of purpose assesses all four of these critical components of the construct.

K. C. Bronk, *Purpose in Life*, DOI 10.1007/978-94-007-7491-9_9,

The reason the beyond-the-self dimension of purpose is missing from existing surveys is likely because it is difficult to design brief survey questions to capture it. First a survey would need to identify an individuals, long-term, personally meaningful aim—if, of course, one exists. Then it would need to determine the degree to which this aim was motivating because of what it would allow the individual to contribute to the world beyond-the-self. Even if a survey item could be designed to capture this motivation, however, it would be difficult to tease apart socially desirable responses from genuine ones. Interviews and diary research circumvent this potential pitfall by offering participants the opportunity to spontaneously broach beyond-the-self concerns. When these concerns arise without prompting, it is more likely that they are genuinely experienced. However interviews are time intensive and costly to conduct and diary methods do not allow for follow-up questions.

Designing a survey, or another inexpensive and efficient measure, that captures all four dimensions of purpose, though difficult, represents a worthwhile activity. Doing so would almost certainly lead to a significant increase in the existing body of empirical research on the construct. Researchers who conduct interviews, investigate diary entries, and review historical documents are limited by small sample sizes, privacy concerns, and incomplete records. These shortcomings could be avoided with a better and more complete measure of purpose.

Longitudinal Investigations

To balance the point in time data generated by survey research, longitudinal research is also needed, especially since purpose is a developmental construct (Damon 2008). A serious exploration of inspiring sources of purpose typically corresponds with the search for identity, beginning during adolescence, taking form during emerging adulthood, and evolving during midlife and later adulthood (Bronk 2011, 2012; Damon 2008; Damon et al. 2003; Deeks and McCabe 2004; Erikson 1968, 1980; Ryff et al. 1996; Ryff and Singer 2008). A purpose in life represents an important life-course plan, and yet rarely has the construct been studied over time to see how it changes and evolves and if indeed plans made during adolescence and emerging adulthood orient individuals into midlife and beyond. Cross-sectional research on purpose is plentiful (e.g. Bronk et al. 2009; Damon 2008; Reker 2005), but only a handful of longitudinal studies have been conducted, and most of these span only a matter of weeks (e.g. Steger et al. 2006) or months (Fahlman et al. 2009; Ryff and Essex 1992; Steger and Kashdan 2007; Steger et al. 2008). At present, only one study has followed youth over five-years, across adolescence and emerging adulthood (Bronk 2011, 2012; Damon 2008). This is an important first step, but certainly not an ending point.

Longitudinal research on purpose could be used to address a variety of important questions. For instance, empirical studies suggest that purpose levels fluctuate following certain experiences and transitions (Bronk 2012; Paloutzian 1981; Ryff and Essex 1992; Ryff et al. 1996; Stillman et al. 2009), but how do purposes change across different stages of life? To what degree does purpose represent a stable trait and to what degree does it represent a fluctuating state? Under what conditions are purposes established during adolescence and emerging adulthood still valid in midlife and late adulthood? How does the continuity or discontinuity of purpose impact well-being?

In addition to answering questions about the stable and enduring nature of purpose and its relation to well-being, longitudinal research should also be conducted to reveal causal relationships relevant to the construct. Much of the research conducted on purpose to date is correlational in nature, and longitudinal studies are needed to establish causal models (Pinquart 2002). This kind of research is time consuming and expensive, but given the central role of purpose in optimal human development, it is warranted.

Investigations of Immoral or Ignoble Purposes

Not only has much of the existing research on purpose been correlational in nature, but it has also been largely limited to noble or moral forms of the construct. A close reading of the definition reveals that the construct need not be positive in nature. Ignoble and immoral forms of purpose certainly exist, and while they may not contribute to optimal well-being in the same way moral aims do, an understanding of these types of purpose is also warranted.

Some may argue that is difficult if not impossible to determine which purposes are moral and which ones are immoral in nature. According to a purely relativistic view, purpose is a social construction and the designation of it as noble or ignoble is a matter of interpretation, varying according to one's cultural or individual perspective. Classification of purposes depends largely on social and political history and on one's construal of the social structure.

While this view has its merit for understanding how historical, environmental, and personal transformations affect purpose and for describing how an understanding of what is considered desirable or good can evolve over time, a more general consensus is that a distinction between moral and immoral purposes is in fact possible. In the social sciences, four approaches to distinguishing between ignoble and noble aims have been used with some regularity. The interested reader is directed to *Exploring the Nature and Development of purpose in Youth: A Consensus Document* (Bronk et al. 2004) for a fuller discussion of each of these approaches.

Assuming we can distinguish noble from ignoble purpose, then it is possible to explore the role of negative purpose, and doing so is necessary to gain a fuller understanding of the entire construct as opposed to only positive manifestations of it. Useful questions to explore regarding negative purposes vary widely, but include the following: what is the experience of leading a life of immoral purpose like? Do ignoble purposes stem from the same sources as positive ones? What are the characteristics of individuals who pursue ignoble aims? What types of early experiences are associated with the development of negative purposes? What types of supports help ignoble purposes thrive, and what kinds of interventions can redirect them?

Learning more about ignoble purposes would not only afford a fuller understanding of the complex and multifaceted purpose construct, but would also shed further light on the relationship between positive purposes and optimal development. If ignoble purposes turn out to be associated with certain aspects of well-being, that would reveal information about which components of positive purposes are related to which aspects of well-being. For instance, like a moral purpose, an immoral purpose provides a personally meaningful, long-term aim, giving one's life direction and focus. It seems likely that the goal-orientation of purpose, whether positive or negative in nature, may be related to certain aspects of well-being, and understanding which ones would reveal the unique contribution of *positive* purposes to optimal health. Beyond providing a fuller understanding of a complex construct and beyond illuminating aspects of positive forms of purpose, it would be important to understand more about negative purposes in order to learn how we might intervene to redirect them to more positive ends.

Role of Negative Experiences

Not only is it worthwhile to learn more about negative purposes, but it is also important to learn more about the role negative life experiences play in the discovery and pursuit of purpose. Dramatic books and movies often portray individuals who lose their sense of purpose when confronted by challenging and disorienting circumstances. But this is not the case for all people. Some individuals persevere toward personally meaningful aims in spite of difficult experiences. Frankl was certainly one of those individuals.

> We must never forget that we may also find meaning in life even when confronted with a hopeless situation, when facing a fate that cannot be changed. For what then matters is to bare witness to the uniquely human potential at its best, which is to transform a personal tragedy into triumph, to turn one's predicament into a human achievement. When we are on longer able to change a situation- just think of an incurable disease such as inoperable cancer- we are challenged to change ourselves (Frankl 1959, p. 135).

Frankl spoke from experience. He maintained his purpose while being held as a prisoner in a Nazi concentration camp. His belief in the importance of meaning and purpose to promoting well-being was refined during an experience of extreme deprivation and suffering. He designed Logotherapy as a therapeutic approach to help all people, including individuals who must endure seemingly meaningless suffering, to discover a purpose for their lives. Frankl was careful to point out that suffering and negative events are not pre-requisites to discovering purpose, but neither are they incompatible with doing so.

Similarly, little research has focused on the role of purpose in suffering. The Meaning in Suffering Test (MIST; Starck 1983, 1985) was designed to assess Frankl's assertion that people can maintain a their purpose even during prolonged periods of unavoidable suffering. However, few empirical studies have employed this measure. In fact, a recent literature review spanning 50 years of research

(1956–2006) was conducted using Medline, PsychInfo, PsychArticles, CINAHL, ProQuest, Ebsco, and MasterFile Premier databases, and the only studies this search generated were ones assessing the measure's validity (Fjelland et al. 2008). Given that the measurement tool appears to have sound psychometric properties (e.g. Schulenberg et al. 2006), and that Frankl highlighted the importance of meaning in suffering, this seems like a significant oversight. As Frankl eloquently noted, purpose may be particularly important to individuals who are suffering. "A man who becomes conscious of the responsibility he bears toward a human being who affectionately waits for him, or an unfinished work, will never be able to throw away life. He knows the 'why' for his existence, and will be able to bear almost any 'how'" (Frankl 1959, p. 101). Frankl strongly believed that having a purpose in life helped individuals endure life's difficult circumstances. A deeper understanding, generated by empirical studies on the topic, would reveal important information about how purpose could be fostered during times of extreme hardship to help ease people's suffering.

According to Frankl, people are not only capable of maintaining purposes under dire circumstances, but they are also likely to discover purposes following negative events in their lives. Few empirical studies have explored ways that negative life events can trigger the growth of personally meaningful aspirations. One such study, a longitudinal investigation of youth purpose exemplars, determined that several of the young people were catapulted to action following disturbing events close to home (Bronk 2012). These preliminary findings, coupled with frequent news stories about individuals who work to change laws and policies following personal, local and national tragedies, suggest that this could be a fruitful line of inquiry. Given the positive role of purpose in optimal well-being (Benson 2006; Bundick 2010; Damon 2008; Gillham et al. 2011; Peterson and Seligman 2004; Ryff and Singer 2008; Seligman 2011) and the relative rarity of discovering purpose (Bronk et al. 2009; Bronk et al. 2010; Damon 2008), exploring the role of potential negative triggers is necessary.

Purpose among Youth From Highly Challenging Backgrounds

Given that purpose appears to alleviate suffering, it would be important to investigate the construct among youth who come from particularly challenging backgrounds. While a small body of research has focused on the role of purpose among individuals suffering from terminal health issues (e.g. Starck 1983, 1985), virtually no research has explored purpose among youth who are homeless or otherwise struggling to meet basic needs. In the midst of fighting for survival, how can these youth manage to find purposes for their lives? What kinds of purposes inspire them? Does finding purpose improve their odds of survival? Does it improve the quality of their lives? Of course, studying purpose among this population is likely to prove very difficult, but these youth may have more to gain from discovering a purpose than most. Accordingly, an investigation would be highly worthwhile. It might be useful to recruit individuals who already work with this population to serve as co-researchers since they are likely to elicit fuller participation given their established relationships with these young people. Working with this special population of youth to help them not only meet their basic needs, but to also think beyond their current circumstances would require great sensitivity and self-awareness. However, Frankl (1959) would likely argue that discovering a purpose, even in these very difficult circumstances, is not only possible but could be live sustaining.

Different Types of Purpose

A wide range of purposes inspire individuals, and much remains to be learned about how these different types of purpose develop and function. As discussed at greater length in Chap. 6 (Inspiring Types of Life Purpose), categorizing purposes can be a difficult task. An emerging adult who plans to become a teacher and work in rural areas because this is where she feels she can do the most good and because a career in teacher will allow her to support her family, could be said to have career, familial, and service-oriented purposes all at once. Classifying purposes into just one category can be difficult. However, that does not mean that this type of research cannot be conducted. It seems logical to categorize purposes as broadly as is warranted given an individual's reported ultimate aims and to explore the aspirations from each of the relevant angles. This means the fictitious profile above could be included in a study of career, familial, *and* service-oriented purposes.

To date, most empirical studies targeting any particular type of long-term aim have focused on the role of religious purposes, and this line of inquiry has yielded a deeper understanding of many of the particularities of religious purpose discussed in greater detail in Chap. 6 (Inspiring Types of Purpose). A similar approach to studying familial, artistic, career, and civic aims is needed since these distinct types of purposes are likely to follow different developmental trajectories, require diverse forms of supports, and encounter particular challenges.

Empirical studies designed to examine distinct kinds of purposes are needed for several reasons. First, it is important to know more about different types of purpose so that effective programs and interventions can be designed to support each one. Second, to fully understand purpose, we need to know how it functions in each of its potential forms. Artistic purposes, for example, are typically focused not on serving individuals or causes, but instead on serving the art form. These purposes clearly differ from civic or service oriented purposes where individuals typically seek to directly impact others, and these aims likely differ from political or religious ones where individuals often work to promote personally meaningful values. What difference does it make, especially with regards to optimal human functioning, when individuals seek to serve an art form rather than a group of individuals, a cause, or a personal value?

On a more fine grained level, it is also worthwhile to explore similarities and differences within a particular area of purposeful pursuit. Empirical studies aimed at exploring different career oriented aims, for example, are needed. Studies should be conducted to determine if certain career paths, such as teaching, nursing, and social work, are more likely than others to inspire purpose. Comparing individuals in particular fields who consider their jobs to be a calling could be compared with individuals in the same field who do not identify their careers as sources of personal meaning. Such findings would yield important insight into the more specific developmental trajectory of a particular type of career-oriented purpose. These findings are also likely to have important implications for secondary and tertiary educational programs, internship opportunities, and career counseling programs. They may even have important policy implications. Clearly much remains to be learned in this vast space.

Cultural and Cross-cultural Studies

In addition to learning more about different types of purposes, it would also be valuable to know more about cultural and ethnic variations purpose. To establish a more complete understanding of what purpose is and how it functions, cross-cultural and cultural studies are needed. Cross-cultural studies examine psychological difference between cultures while cultural studies focus on differences within a culture (King et al. in press). To better understand which aspects of the purpose construct are universal and which ones are culturally specific, and to gain a fuller understanding of the way personal aspirations develop among a wider array of individuals, both of these research approaches should be applied to the study of purpose.

Cultural studies of purpose to date have primarily been limited to the United States, and only a few cross-cultural studies of purpose exist. Several measures of purpose and closely related constructs have been translated into different languages (e.g. Japanese Purpose in Life test, J-PIL; Okado 1998; Chinese Purpose in Life test, C-PIL; Shek et al. 1987; Japanese Meaning in Life Questionnaire, JMLQ; Steger et al. 2008), but they have rarely been administered. The handful of cross-cultural studies that have been conducted have largely focused on comparing the prevalence of purpose among individuals from one country with the prevalence of purpose among similarly aged individuals in the United States (e.g. Shek et al. 1987; Steger et al. 2008). Results of this line of inquiry conclude that purpose and meaning are more prevalent in the United States than in many Eastern cultures (e.g. Korean versus Americans—Hauser et al. 1992; Chinese versus Americans—Shek et al. 1987; Japanese versus Americans—Steger et al. 2008) and that striving for meaning is more prevalent in Eastern culture than it is in America (Steger et al. 2008). Researchers believe this discrepancy may be due to the fact that independent cultures, such as the United States, emphasize the self as an individual agent (Heine et al. 2001). Individuals in these cultures are encouraged to establish and maintain positive feelings about themselves, (Heine et al. 2001), and the presence of meaning and purpose is strongly associated with positive Feelings (King et al. 2006) and well-being (Seligman 2002; Zika and Chamberlain 1987; Gillham et al. 2011). Alternately, individuals in interdependent cultures view themselves as members of communal and social networks, and they are encouraged to strive for self-improvement (Heine et al. 1999; Oishi and Diener 2003). They tend to be more concerned with process than outcomes; accordingly, searching for meaning makes sense in these cultures. These preliminary findings suggest, as would be expected, that important cultural differences around the nature of purpose exist and underscore the need for additional cross-cultural studies of the construct.

More cultural studies are also needed. The vast majority of research on purpose to date has taken place in autonomous, Western cultures (e.g. Crumbaugh and Maholick 1964; Damon 2008; Ryff and Singer 1998). The limited scope of this research has undoubtedly curtailed our understanding of the full construct. Little empirical evidence is available that illuminates the nature and forms of purpose in cultures that ascribe to an ethic of community or an ethic of divinity (Shweder 2003). Presumably purposes in these cultures are more focused on responsibility to family and community or fidelity to one's faith or religious beliefs, respectively. Because these cultures encourage a sense of duty to others, either communal or sacred others, rather than a sense of responsibility to the self, it seems likely that beyond-the-self aims and self-oriented aims are more closely aligned in these cultures (Bronk et al. 2004), but the potential impact of this on the development, prevalence, or role of purpose is as of yet unknown.

Additionally, in some cultures, life commitments are pre-determined for youth. Rather than choosing the path they hope to pursue, young people in these cultures are prepared for particular roles. How does this impact the nature of purpose? Presumably, the incorporation of a purpose into one's sense of identity is more continuous in these cultures than in Western cultures, where young people have to discover for themselves a purpose for their lives. These different orientations are also reflected in rites of passages. In the contemporary United States, and many Western cultures, rites of passage are relatively rare, but those that exist tend to focus on encouraging youth to gain self-confidence and self-knowledge (Bronk et al. 2004). In other cultures, rites of passage ceremonies mark the young person's entrance into adult and communal roles. How do cultural practices and expectations in interdependent cultures impact the development of purpose among young people?

This discussion of potential cultural differences is very cursory. It is not intended to serve as an overview of all or even most of the potentially important cultural differences that exist with regards to purpose. It is only meant to highlight the need for more cultural and cross-cultural studies of the construct.

Physical Benefits of Purpose

Another area where additional empirical research is warranted is around the potential physical benefits of leading a life of purpose. Research in this area is still in its infancy, but early findings are promising. As discussed in greater detail in Chap. 3 (The Role of Purpose in Optimal Human Functioning), high rates of purpose are associated with a variety of positive health indicators, including improved cardiovascular health (Ryff et al. 2004). Individual with purpose are less likely to suffer from Alzheimer's Disease, mild cognitive impairment (Boyle et al. 2010), and chronic pain (Kass et al. 1991). In fact, two studies have concluded that individuals with purpose tend to live longer than individuals without purpose (Boyle et al. 2009; Krause 2009).

Though the association between purpose and indicators of positive health is consistent, it is modest. Additionally, only a handful of studies have explored the relationship between purpose and physical well-being, and most of the few studies that have are correlational in nature. Given the promising early findings, additional investigation into the role of purpose in physical health is needed. Beyond conducting correlational studies, researchers should carry out longitudinal research to test possible causal relationships. Does purpose contribute to physical health, or are people who are physically healthy more inclined to discover personally meaningful aims, or is a third variable responsible for both high rates of purpose and physical health? Additional research in this area is needed.

Support for the Development of Purpose

Lastly, given that having a life purpose is consistently associated with positive physical (e.g. Ryff et al. 2004) and psychological health (Bronk 2008; Bronk et al. 2009; Damon 2008) and given that only a relatively small percentage of young people commit to purposes (Bronk et al. 2009; Damon 2008; Bronk et al. 2010), additional empirical research into how to support and foster the development of purpose is called for. Chapter 5 (Origins of and Supports for Purpose) synthesizes existing research regarding effective approaches for cultivating personally meaningful aspirations. A series of studies outlined in greater detail in Chap. 5 conclude that relatively straightforward interventions can significantly impact the likelihood that young people will discover a purpose for their lives (e.g. Bundick 2011; Dik et al. 2011; Pizzolato et al. 2011). This conclusion should encourage us to learn more. Other than these few intervention studies, most of the research on how to support the development of purpose is theoretical and based on studies of related topics. Theoretical findings largely dovetail with the available empirical results, which suggests that purpose functions in expected ways, but empirical research focused directly on the construct is still needed, especially in particular settings.

For example, empirical studies should investigate ways that parents can help foster purpose at home. Surprisingly, few empirical studies focus on this topic directly. Theoretical research suggests that parents should encourage their children and adolescents to reflect on their personal values, develop a language for discussing purposes, and focus on far-horizon rather than short-horizon (Damon 2008; Fry 1998). Parents should also share their own purposes with their children (Damon 2008) and encourage their children to thoughtfully engage in a few potentially purposeful activities to reveal where young people's interests and talents lie (Bronk 2012; Shamah 2011). While these approaches offer a useful starting point for parents, empirical work is needed to clarify how each of these recommendations works in practice, to confirm and extend these recommended steps, and to determine if other, perhaps even more effective strategies, exist.

Additional empirical research in schools would also be useful. Schools are one of the few areas where any empirical research on supporting purpose has been conducted, and existing studies suggest that there are a variety of steps teachers, administrators, and coaches can take to increase the likelihood that students will discover meaningful purposes for their lives (e.g. Dik et al. 2011; Pizzolato et al. 2011). However, existing studies largely reflect add-on approaches to fostering purpose. In other words, they feature additional conversations, activities, and interventions designed to cultivate discussions of and reflections on purpose. Given that many teachers and administrators already feel overburdened by the myriad of add-on programs currently in place, it seems unlikely that additional programs and requirements of this sort will be well received on a broader level. Beyond this, one-time interventions are somewhat limited in their effectiveness. Ideally, purpose-fostering activities would infuse secondary and tertiary school cultures. They would represent on-going, school-wide efforts rather than one-time activities. But what would this look like in practice, and how should it be carried out? Empirical studies designed to determine how to build a culture of purpose within a school setting are needed.

Career and college counseling sessions represent appropriate school-based venues for deep discussions of purpose. One empirical study revealed that a relatively brief career counseling intervention significantly increased rates of purpose among students considering different professional paths (Dik et al. 2011). Much work remains to be done in this area though, as empirical studies are needed to determine how to most effectively help students identify and incorporate their personally meaningful aims in to their plans for their future. Evaluations of existing programs are also needed to identify if and how they support the development of students' personally meaningful aims.

The mentoring relationship is another important element to consider with regards to purpose development. Empirical studies of purpose find that, among other variables, having close, long-term relationships with mentors distinguishes most youth with purpose from many youth without (Bronk 2008). Adults who share youths' passions can serve as important mentors providing critical support, guidance, and encouragement (Bronk 2012; Parks 2011), and they can help youth reflect on their purposes (Bundick 2011; Fry 1998; Pizzolato et al. 2011). However, not much is known about how youth seeking purpose typically encounter mentors nor is much known about how mentors should effectively interact with youth around their personally meaningful life aims. What kinds of conversations are particularly useful? How should adults reach out to youth who clearly have a purpose, but who are shy or socially awkward? Is there a systematic approach for matching youth with mentors help youth discover and remain committed to a purpose over time? What kinds of conversations are likely to elicit thoughtful reflections on youths purposes? More research is needed about mentors and other potential sources of social support for the development of purpose.

Largely as a result of Frankl's (1959) book on the topic, Ryff's research on psychological well-being (Ryff and Keyes 1995; Ryff and Singer 1998), and the growth of positive psychology, psychological attention on the purpose construct has increased significantly. In the past fifteen years in particular, the number of empirical studies and theoretical papers focused on the purpose construct has increased substantially. Studies have focused on a wide range of important issues relevant to purpose, and together they have provided a solid understanding of the nature and prevalence of purpose, its forms, its roles across the lifespan, and its associations with optimal human functioning. However, psychological consideration of this important construct is still a relatively new phenomenon, and clearly more work is needed to generate a fuller understanding of the benefits of leading a life of purpose.

At the same time, it is also important to explore the limits of purpose. Though the construct is associated with a wide range of positive outcomes, at least in some cases, it is not associated with happiness, and this line of inquiry begins to highlight the construct's limitations. Like any psychological concept, purpose has limits—there is no singular construct that can cure all ills for all people under all circumstances—and additional empirical investigations are needed that shed light not only on what the potential is for purpose, but also on what its limitations are. When we fully understand both of these issues, we will be much better prepared to provide empirically-based guidance to people seeking purpose for their lives.

References

Benson, P. L. (2006). *All kids are our kids: What communities must do to raise caring and responsible children and adolescents (2nd ed.)* San Francisco: Jossey-Bass.

Boyle, P. A., Barnes, L. L., Buchman, A. S., & Bennett, D. A. (2009). Purpose in life is associated with mortality among community-dwelling older persons. *Psychosomatic medicine, 71*(5), 574–579.

Boyle, P. A., Barnes, L. L., Buchman, A. S., & Bennett, D. A. (2010). Effect of a Purpose in life on risk of incident Alzheimer Disease and mild cognitive impairment in community-dwelling older persons. *Archives of General Psychiatry, 67*(3), 304–310. doi:10.1001/archgenpsychiatry.2009.208.

Bronk, K. C. (2011). Portraits of purpose: The role of purpose in identity formation. A special issue on Instructing for and Supporting Youth Purpose in. *New Directions in Youth Development, 132,* 31–44.

Bronk, K. C. (2012). A grounded theory of youth purpose. *Journal of Adolescent Research, 27,* 78–109. http://dx.doi.org/10.1177/0743558411412958.

Bronk, K. C., Hill, P., Lapsley, D. K., Talib, T., & Finch, W. H. (2009). Purpose, hope, and life satisfaction in three age groups. *Journal of Positive Psychology, 4*(6), 500–510.

Bronk, K. C., Menon, J. L., & Damon, W. (2004). *Youth purpose: Conclusions from a working conference of leading scholars*. John Templeton Foundation Press.

Bronk, K. C., Finch, W. H., & Talib, T. (2010). The prevalence of a purpose in life among high ability adolescents. *High Ability Studies, 21*(2), 133–145.

Bundick, M. (2011). The benefits of reflecting on and discussing purpose in life in emerging adulthood. *New Directions for Youth Development, 132,* 89–103.

Bundick, M. J., Yeager, D. S., King, P. E., & Damon, W. (2010). Thriving across the lifespan. In R. M. Lerner, M. E. Lamb, A. M. Freund, & W. F. Overton (Eds.), *Handbook of life- span development, Vol. 1: Cognition, Biology and Methods* (pp. 882–923). Hoboken, NJ: John Wiley & Sons.

Crumbaugh, J. C., & Maholick, L. T. (1964). An experimental study in existentialism: The psychometic approach to Frankl's concept of noogenic neurosis. *Journal of Clinical Psychology, 20,* 200–207.

Damon, W. (2008). *The path to purpose: Helping our children find their calling in life*. New York: The Free Press.

Damon, W., Menon, J., & Bronk, K. C. (2003). The development of purpose during adolescence. *Applied Developmental Science, 7*(3), 119–128.

Deeks, A. A., & McCabe, M. P. (2004). Well-being and menopause: An investigation of purpose in life, self-acceptance, and social role in premenopausal, perimenopausal, and post menopausal women. *Quality of Life Research, 13,* 389–398.

Dik, B. J., Steger, M. F., Gibson, A., & Peisner, W. (2011). Make Your Work Matter: Development and pilot evaluations of a purpose-centered career education intervention. *New Directions for Youth Development, 132,* 59–73.

Erikson, E. H. (1968). *Identity: youth and crisis*. New York: W. W. Norton.

Erikson, E. H. (1980). *Identity and the life cycle (paperback)*. New York: W.W. Norton & Company Inc.

Fahlman, S. A., Merce, K. B., Gaskovski, P., Eastwood, A. E., & Eastwood, J. D. (2009). Does a lack of life meaning cause boredom? Results from psychometric, longitudinal and experimental analyses. *Journal of Social and Clinical Psychology, 28*(3), 307–340.

Fjelland, J. E., Barron, C. R., & Foxall, M. (2008). A review of instruments measuring two aspects of meaning: search for meaning and meaning in illness. *Journal of Advanced Nursing, 62*(4), 394–406.

Frankl, V. E. (1959). *Man's search for meaning*. New York: Simon & Schuster.

Fry, P. S. (1998). The development of personal meaning and wisdom in adolescence: A reexamination of moderating and consolidating factors and influences. In P. T. P. Wong (Ed.), *The human quest for meaning: A handbook of psychological research and clinical applications (2nd ed)* (pp. 91–110). New York: Routledge.

Gillham, J., Adams-Deutsch, Z., Werner, J., Reivich, K., Coulter-Heindl, V., Linkins, M., Winder, B., Peterson, C., Park, N., Abenavoli, R., Contero, A., & Seligman, M. E. P. (2011). Character Strengths Predict Subjective Well-Being during Adolescence. *Journal of Positive Psychology, 6*(1), 31–44. doi:10.1080/17439760.2010.53677..

Hauser, R. M., Sewell, W. H., Logan, J. A., Hauser, T. S., Ryff, C., Caspi, A., & MacDonald, M. (1992). The Wisconsin Longitudinal Study: Adults as Parents and Children at Age 50. *CDE Working Paper 92–02*. Madison, WI: Center for Demography and Ecology.

Heine, S. J., Kitayama, S., & Lehman, D. R. (2001). Cultural differences in self-evaluation: Japanese readily accept negative self-relevant information. *Journal of Cross-Cultural Psychology, 32,* 434–443.

Kass, J. D., Friedman, R., Leserman, J., Caudill, M., Zuttermeister, P. C., & Benson, H. (1991). An inventory of positive psychological attitudes with potential relevance to health outcomes: Validation and preliminary testing. *Behavioral Medicine, 17*(3), 121–129.

King, L. A., Hicks, J. A., & Krull, J., & Del Gaiso, A. K. (2006). Positive affect and the experience of meaning in life. *Journal of Personality and Social Psychology, 90,* 179–196.

Krause, N. (2009). Meaning in life and mortality. *The Journals of Gerontology Series B: Psychological Sciences and Social Sciences, 64B*(4), 517–527. DOI:10.1093/geronb/gbp047.

Oishi, S., & Diener, E. (2003). Culture and well-beng: The cycle of action, evaluation, and decision. *Personality and Social Psychology Bulletin, 29,* 939–949.

Okado, T. (1998). *The Japanese version of the Purpose in Life Test*. Tokyo: System Publica.

Paloutzian, R. F. (1981). Purpose in life and value changes following conversion. *Journal of Personality and Social Psychology, 41*(6), 1153–1160.

Peterson, C., & Seligman, M. E. P. (2004). *Character strengths and virtues: A handbook and classification*. New York: Oxford University Press.

Pinquart, M. (2002). Creating and maintaining purpose in life in old age: A meta-analysis. *Ageing International, 27*(2), 90–114.

Pizzolato, J. E., Brown, E. L., & Kanny, M. A. (2011). Purpose plus: Supporting youth purpose, control, and academic achievement. *New Directions for Youth Development, 132,* 75–88.

Reker, G. T. (2005). Meaning in life of young, middle-aged, and older adults: Factorial validity, age, and gender invariance of the Personal Meaning Index (PMI). *Personality and Individual Differences, 38,* 71–85.

Ryff, C., & Essex, M. J. (1992). The interpretation of life experience and well-being: The sample case of relocation. *Psychology and Aging, 7*(4), 507–517.

Ryff, C. D., & Keyes, C. L. (1995). The Structure of psychological well- being revisited. *Journal of Personality and Social Psychology, 69*(4), 719–27.

Ryff, C., & Singer, B. (1998). The contours of positive human health. *Psychological Inquiry, 9*(1), 1–28.

Ryff, C. D., & Singer, B. H. (2008). Know thyself and become what you are: A eudaimonic approach to psychological well-being. *Journal of Happiness Studies, 9,* 13–39.

Ryff, C., Schmutte, P. S., & Lee, Y. H. (1996). How children turn out: Implications for parental self-evaluation. In C. D. Ryff, & M. M. Seltzer (Eds.), *The parental experience in midlife* (pp. 383–422). Chicago: University of Chicago Press.

Ryff, C. D., Singer, B., & Love, G. D. (2004). Positive health: Connecting well-being with biology. *Philosophical Transactions: Biological Sciences, 359,* 1383–1394.

Schulenberg, S. E., Gohm, C. L., Anderson, C. (2006). The Meaning in Suffering Test (MIST): A unitary or multidimensional measure? *International Forum for Logotherapy, 29*(2), 103–106.

Seligman, M. E. P. (2002). *Authentic happiness: Using the new positive psychology to realize your potential for lasting fulfillment.* New York, NY: Free Press.

Seligman, M. E. P. (2011). *Flourishing: New York: A visionary new understanding of happiness and well-being.* New York: Free Press.

Shamah, D. (2011). Supporting a strong sense of purpose: Lessons from a rural community. *New Directions for Youth Development, 132,* 45–58.

Shek, D. T., Hong, E. W., & Cheung, M. Y. P. (1987). The purpose in life questionnaire in a Chinese context. *Journal of Psychology, 121*(1), 77–83.

Shweder, R. A. (2003). *Why do men barbecue? Recipes for cultural psychology.* Cambridge, MA: Harvard University Press.

Starck, P. L. (1983). Patients' perceptions of the meaning of suffering. *The International Forum for Logotherapy, 6,* 110–116.

Starck, P. L. (1985). *Guidelines—Meaning in Suffering Test.* Berkeley, CA: Institute of Logotherapy Press.

Steger, M. F., Frazier, P., Oishi, S., & Kaler, M. (2006). The Meaning in Life Questionnaire: Assessing the presence of and search for meaning in life. *Journal of Counseling Psychology, 53,* 80–93.

Steger, M. F., & Kashdan, T. B. (2007). Stability and specificity of meaning in life and life satisfaction over one year. *Journal of Happiness Studies, 8,* 161–179.

Steger, M. F., Kawabata, Y., Shimai, S., & Otake, K. (2008). The meaningful life in Japan and the United States: Levels and correlates of meaning in life. *Journal of Research in Personality, 42,* 660–678.

Stillman, T. F., Baumeister, R. F., Lambert, N., Crescioni, A. W., DeWall, C. N., & Fincham, F. D. (2009). Alone and without purpose: Life loses meaning following social exclusion. *Journal of Experimental Social Psychology, 45,* 686–94.

MIX
Papier aus verantwortungsvollen Quellen
Paper from responsible sources
FSC® C105338

If you have any concerns about our products,
you can contact us on
ProductSafety@springernature.com

In case Publisher is established outside the EU,
the EU authorized representative is:
Springer Nature Customer Service Center GmbH
Europaplatz 3, 69115 Heidelberg, Germany

Printed by Libri Plureos GmbH
in Hamburg, Germany